Always with Children

by

Mary Aston

DORRANCE PUBLISHING CO., INC.
PITTSBURGH, PENNSYLVANIA 15222

ISBN # 0-8059-4053-7
Printed in the United States of America

First Printing

For information or to order additional books, please write:
Dorrance Publishing Co., Inc.
643 Smithfield Street
Pittsburgh, Pennsylvania 15222
U.S.A.

Dedication

*To my mother for her
constant love and encouragement.*

Table of Contents

Acknowledgements

A big thank you to all my family, colleagues, friends and of course the children for making this book possible.

Chapter 1

BEGINNINGS

For as long as I can remember I have loved children, especially babies. As a child I would spend hours playing with my dolls; I would take them for walks in a pram, dress and undress them and brush their hair. When I pretended to be a mother, was I perhaps preparing to become a children's nurse?

In 1945, when I was nine years old, my sister, Pamela, and brother, Peter, were eighteen and sixteen, respectively. The war was over, and we all returned to live in my father's vicarage at Guildford. He had been an army padre in prisoner-of-war camps in Germany for the past five years. During the war my mother had taken us to Cornwall and Devon.

In time we were together again as a family. As the vicar's wife, my mother organised meetings for young wives in the parish. My best friend, Gill, and I used to love looking after the toddlers; we played with them in the nursery while their mothers attended the meeting in the sitting room opposite.

In Guildford, I went to a local girls' day school and made a lot of friends. In Devon I had been a weekly boarder, as there was no school close enough for me to go daily. This school had been evacuated for the duration of the war. It was now wonderful to live at home with both my parents and go to a day school. The next three years were very happy. I had exciting birthday parties and invited my friends for tea and games. My parents were exceptionally good at organising children. We often wore fancy dress. The dining room was large; we could seat about fourteen chairs with a server round the mahogany table. My mother provided a wonderful spread and, as always, my favourite wobbly jellies and a cake.

In those days there was not much traffic, and my friends and I used to go off on long bicycle rides taking picnics with us. Swimming at the local Guildford lido was also popular. I was forever demanding a sixpence after school so that I could go swimming with my friends. I could be very adventurous. I remember one evening in particular. When I was about ten, a fair came to a park just down the road from our house. Sometimes a couple living in a flat in the vicarage would baby-sit when both my parents were out. Once I was tucked up in bed, they would occasionally come up to see me. I was desperate to see the fairground lit up at night. When all was quiet and I knew my parents had gone out, I slipped on a warm coat and a pair of shoes, tiptoed down the stairs and out of the house, then ran all the way to the fair. It was a fantastic sight! When my favourite roundabout stopped, I leapt up on to the nearest horse and clung tightly to the pole. Soon we were going round and round and up and down to the sound of the hurdy-gurdy music. The ride was magical. As soon as the music and ride ended, I ran back home and slipped back into bed, delighted by this successful adventure. It was a very long time before I told anyone what I had done.

Since my sister was training to be a physical education teacher at Dartford College and my brother had just joined the army, most of the time I was the only one at home. When I was eleven years old, I became a boarder at Sherborne School for girls in Dorset. I was not academic but loved all sports. I can honestly say that those years were happy, and I made some lifelong friends.

During the last year at Sherborne I was games captain. Every day each of the sixty girls in my house had to be allocated to a game of hockey, lacrosse or netball. The lists would be read out at lunch and then shown to the house mistress. I was responsible for choosing and coaching the house teams. I was incredibly keen that we should win the inter-house cups. One evening our headmistress came to supper, and she was amazed when I told her that the hockey first team was to practise at 7.00 A.M. before the finals that afternoon. It was worth the effort, as we won the cup that term.

I left school with five "O" levels at the end of the summer term in 1954. Now I had to consider seriously what I would do with my life. For some reason the school staff had encouraged me to take up training for orthoptics, and I had been accepted at both Moorfields and Oxford eye hospitals. It was assumed that I would start at one of these hospitals to learn about the treatment and care of children's squints.

To celebrate the end of my school days, my mother and I spent ten fabulous days at the Edinburgh festival. We went to the Tattoo, concerts and plays and visited many exhibitions. But I felt distinctly uneasy about the future. Did I really want to spend the rest of my working life looking at children's squints? The answer was no.

I discussed the problem with my mother. She was amazingly understanding. I then wrote to both training schools and politely turned down the places offered. I decided that I would much rather work on a children's ward in a hospital.

An appointment was made for me to see the matron of the Salisbury Infirmary, and my mother accompanied me to the interview. We sat side by side on high-backed chairs in front of a large mahogany desk; on the other side sat the matron. She was very impressive, immediately commanding my attention and respect. She wore a spotless navy-blue uniform with badges pinned on her left breast, and a high, complicated white starched cap sat on her greying hair. She had a kind, intelligent face.

"Why do you want to work with children in a hospital?" she asked. I must have sounded very young and inexperienced; however, my enthusiasm must have impressed her. She admitted that she did require an orderly to work on the children's surgical ward at Odstock Hospital, which was affiliated with the Salisbury Infirmary. I would sleep in the nurses' home at the infirmary and go to Odstock each morning on the hospital bus in order to start work at 7.00.

The matron explained that it was the first time she had employed an orderly with a public school education, but she was willing to give me a trial because I was so keen to have the job. So it was arranged that I would start the following Monday, which was less than a week away. A uniform would be made for me and would be ready on my arrival at the nurses' home on Sunday evening.

The prospect of starting work so soon was exciting. My mother and I spent the next few days shopping, packing and generally preparing for my new life. My mother was, as always, most encouraging. On that Sunday afternoon she drove me the thirty miles to the nurses' home in Salisbury.

An elderly, retired nurse welcomed me and took me to my room on Sunday evening. There was an iron bedstead and well-worn mattress made up with hospital linen, a cupboard, a chest of drawers and a small table and chair. Having been at boarding school, I knew the room would look more like home once I had unpacked my pictures, ornaments and photographs. I discovered my uniform was ready as had been promised.

After a few minutes my mother prepared to leave. We both found saying good-bye difficult. She was going home to an empty house. The strain of being a prisoner of war for five years had been too much for my father, who had died while I was away at school in Dorset. My sister was now married and living abroad, and my brother was in the army stationed in Germany.

Feeling rather alone and a bit scared in my new surroundings, I unpacked and then made my way to the dining room for supper. From then on everyone I met was most friendly and helpful. I went to bed feeling excited at the prospect of seeing the children's ward the next morning.

Fortunately, my alarm clock worked. I leapt out of bed feeling rather apprehensive. My green uniform dress with black webbing belt fitted very well, much to my relief. I put on my newly acquired black stockings and shoes, attached the white linen cap to my hair and wrapped the navy cloak with scarlet lining round my shoulders. I glanced at myself in the mirror and was quite surprised at how smart I looked; then I made my way to the dining room for a quick breakfast before catching the bus to Odstock.

After the war Odstock Hospital, which was built on a hill, became famous as a burns and plastic surgery unit for war casualties. There were rows of long Nissen huts on either side of a long concrete corridor. I was directed down this corridor to the third hut on the left, the children's surgical ward.

Sister Dwyer came forward to greet me. She was middle aged, very tall, slim and efficient looking. She was, in fact, a most experienced and highly regarded paediatric sister. In the ward of twenty-four cots and beds, I could sense a happy, comfortable atmosphere. There was laughter and chatter, children in dressing gowns and slippers were moving freely in the ward, and no one looked scared, though a few more seriously ill children were lying on their beds.

The first job was to clean the ward. The children were asked to climb on to their beds, after which we pushed them and their lockers first to one side and then to the other; the empty floor space was then sprinkled with wet tea leaves and swept. The children thought our work was a great game. A team of about six of us soon had the floor clean and all the furniture damp dusted. Next, the children were washed. Some had a blanket bath, while others were taken to the bathroom. At about nine-thirty the two part-time staff nurses arrived. They were both married and had their own children. During my year at Odstock, they taught me much about caring for children in a hospital. My duties were fairly basic: doing potty rounds; giving out meals; helping to feed the younger children; making beds and cots; fetching medicines from the pharmacy; and carrying specimens to the laboratory for Sister Dwyer and the staff nurses.

On my first day I shadowed a student nurse. I was very weary when I returned to the nurses' home at 5.00 P.M. and climbed the stairs to my room. That night I sleepwalked for the first time. I woke to find myself pushing my bed backwards and forwards across the room. But as I grew used to the routine, I gained more confidence. I can still remember the thrill of receiving my first pay packet.

I went home most weekends to see my mother, but occasionally I stayed in Salisbury for my days off. Once a month a group of us would go to dances at the town hall on a Saturday night. I was always painfully shy, but I remember making some friends and quite enjoyed these occasions.

With this newfound freedom, however, came definite doubts about my religious beliefs. As a vicar's daughter, I had always gone to church, and on Sundays at boarding school, but I had not really thought much about religion before. So while I was in Salisbury, I went to many church services: Plymouth Brethren, Four Square, Jehovah's Witnesses, Baptist and Methodist. In time I came back to the Church of England and attended services in the cathedral, which I came to love.

Many children came to the children's ward at Odstock. One particular child who was about two years old we nicknamed "Noddy". He came from a local gypsy camp and was admitted with terrible gangrene of the toes; two on his right foot had already fallen off, and the others looked very black. We all loved this plucky little character, and with expert treatment and a lot of loving care we managed to save three toes on each foot. His general condition was poor, so he stayed in the hospital for about two months before returning to his gypsy life.

Another child that I remember was a five-year-old girl in the burns unit. She had been standing by an open fire in her home when a spark had caught the material alight. Sometimes I was asked to go and help with her dressings if the unit was short staffed. She had terrible burns down her back and legs. I can remember the terror on her little face as the nurses renewed the dressings. The nurses did all they could to lessen the pain, and I would hold her hands and try to soothe her or distract her with a story. I think I helped the nurses about five times during the four months she was in the hospital. The day before the girl left she asked me to go and say good-bye. The grafts had taken, and all her burns had healed. She was badly scarred, but the pain and terror had gone. It was a very happy day for us all when she was discharged.

I was nearing the end of my first year on the children's ward at the Odstock Hospital. Without realising it I was doing more and more responsible jobs, such as helping with dressings, taking simple stitches out and escorting children to the operating theatre.

One afternoon, when we were not very busy and both staff nurses were on duty, they asked me to go into the sister's office for a chat. They asked what my future plans were. I replied that I had not thought much about the future, as I was so happy at Odstock on the children's ward. They suggested that I should apply to Great Ormond Street Hospital for Sick Children, London, to do my sick children's nurse training.

I applied, and to my amazement I was accepted for the July 1956 course, provided that I acquired an "O" level in mathematics. I decided to leave Odstock to go home and start evening classes for maths at the local education centre. The matron at Great Ormond Street had also advised me to work as a "mother's help" with a normal child in a family for a few months.

Home for me was now in Winchester, as my mother had moved house. I soon found just the job I was looking for. A family in a village about two miles from Winchester had advertised for a mother's help. I applied and was asked to go for an interview. There were two teenage children and Timmy, who was eighteen months old. His mother was finding it difficult to give him and the older children enough individual attention and thought it might help if she had a live-in help from Monday to Friday for a few months. I got the job and started almost immediately.

Timmy was a normal toddler. His mother taught me everything there was to know about looking after a toddler at home, for instance, the importance of a good routine, dressing a child according to the weather, general hygiene practices and prevention of nappy rash. Together we potty-trained Timmy. I helped with everything in the house, the washing, the cleaning of the playroom and Timmy's bedroom, simple cooking and playing with Timmy. We usually went for a walk in the afternoons, and sometimes I took him to birthday parties or just out to tea with his friends.

For some reason mathematics had been my worst subject all through my school years and I failed my examinations. I could not really see why was it so necessary for me to have "O" level maths before starting to train as a children's nurse. Later, I discovered it was an essential qualification, as one had to work out minute doses for injections.

I struggled on with night school classes, and I eventually took the examination again. I passed, much to my relief. By this time Timmy was nearly two and a half and had started going to the village toddlers' group twice a week. His mother seemed more able to cope, so I left only a few weeks before I was due to start my sick children's training at Great Ormond Street.

Chapter 2
MY FIRST YEAR AT GREAT ORMOND STREET HOSPITAL

The eagerly awaited day in July 1956 arrived at last. Twenty-seven of us met in the spacious sitting room of the Great Ormond Street nurses' home behind the main hospital. We stood around in little groups with families and friends, none of us knowing quite what we had let ourselves in for.

After enjoying the tea provided for us, there was a hush. The door opened, and in came the matron. Everyone stood up to let her pass; it was as if the "queen" had entered the room. From the start it was obvious that she was in charge; her nurses were expected to be loyal, polite, caring and hardworking. Throughout our training we were continually reminded how fortunate we were to have been chosen from hundreds of applicants. The matron made all of this clear in her short speech. After she had left the room we all felt very small, even apprehensive.

However, we were soon ushered out to a coach parked outside the nurses' home. Our luggage was stowed as we said farewell to families and friends. Soon we were on our way to the Brook General Hospital, Woolwich, were all GOS nurses spent their first three months training.

At Brook General Hospital, we found that rooms opened off a long, dark corridor on the ground floor. We each had our own room, in alphabetical order, so initially we became acquainted and made friends with girls whose names were nearest to our own. Our uniforms were in our rooms: specially made pink-and-white striped dresses and white starched aprons and caps.

We were a mixed bunch from all over the British Isles; there was also one African girl. We soon became great friends, and I still keep in touch with several of my GOS set. The initial training in the Preliminary Training School (PTS) took place in part of the Brook General Hospital. We had lectures in a classroom, and we used a practical room for first aid and other subjects. We were woken by a bell at 7.30 A.M. and were in uniform until the end of lectures at 5.30 P.M. Saturday and Sunday were free, and many of us went home if we could afford it.

From the first day of training we were paid a salary, but by the time board and lodging were deducted only some eleven pounds a month was left. We spent one day each week on a ward or department at Great Ormond Street. This day in the hospital gave us our first proper insight into what lay ahead.

Although it was a shock to see how terribly sick some of the children were, we also discovered that Great Ormond Street Hospital was essentially a friendly, cheerful place. Parents were welcome to visit at all times. There were bright pictures on the walls and plenty of toys for all ages. Any child who was not too sick was encouraged to be up and about, and school and art classes were available for older children.

Each ward and department had its own sister. Not only did she organise the nursing and care of the children, but each sister taught us about her specialty, such as the heart, skin or head injuries. Each week we returned tired but exhilarated from these practical days.

Many subjects were covered in the classroom at PTS: children's normal anatomy, normal development of children, infectious diseases, diet and its importance in childhood, first aid, and the prevention of accidents.

The last week of PTS was traumatic. In order to move on to the main training we had to pass an examination in every subject. My friend Veronica and I decided to revise together, going over and over the next exam subject late into the night. It paid off, for both Veronica and I passed all subjects, and to my amazement I came second in anatomy. Only one girl failed and had to leave. Breathing a sigh of relief, the rest of us went home for a long weekend break. On our return we were given a room in the large nurses' home on Guildford Street.

One or two of us had started our training with steady boyfriends. Arthur, my boyfriend, was faithful and wrote regularly from Ceylon, where he worked on a tea plantation. We students, however, soon discovered there was little opportunity to have much social life, for we were either too tired or never had the right time off. Also, our conversation tended to become limited to what had just occurred on our ward. Maybe that is why several of my GOS friends have never married and why I married in my thirties.

On the ground floor of the nurses' home there was a large dining room, where all nurses had their meals. Next to it was a long sitting room. There was a separate, panelled dining room for the sisters. A receptionist took telephone messages for us and answered any queries. Post was put into pigeonholes for us to collect. Discipline was strict in the nurses' home; at 11.00 P.M. the main door was locked, though late passes could be obtained on special request. Several West End theatres would donate complimentary tickets to the London teaching hospitals. I remember wonderful evenings at Drury Lane, Covent Garden and The Albert Hall.

I was assigned to the acute surgical ward, called 1C. There were four cubicles down one side for babies or very sick children, and at the end there was a mini-ward with six cots or beds. This assignment was an exciting start for me, for most of the admissions were emergencies. Many children were flown from other children's hospitals in Britain, and some even came from overseas. Babies born with congenital deformities were transferred to us very quickly after birth in order to give them a greater chance of survival.

Like the other junior nurses on the ward, I was allotted basic tasks; if we were on the early shift, we went on duty at 7.30 A.M. and were given a detailed report on each child. From the start we learnt it was essential to be able to observe and to pay close attention to detail. My responsibility was the sluice, which I had to keep clean and tidy at all times. There were two large sterilizers, which I had to fill with water and boil. I dreaded being interrupted by the sister or staff nurse while I was in the middle of this process. I invariably forgot the tap was running and returned to the sluice to find a terrible flood. I then had to turn out all the dirty linen from the skip and quickly clean up the mess before any of my superiors discovered the fiasco.

The nearest I got to the desperately ill babies on the IC ward was when I did the locker round. A locker beside each child had to be emptied and cleaned every day. The nurse on locker round changed towels, flannels and bibs for fresh ones, and restocked the cupboard with nappies and clean clothes. I had to be extremely careful, because there were tubes and bottles and monitors everywhere, and in the cubicles I had to wear a mask and gown.

I was on IC for three months, and then my set changed wards. I went to a medical ward, 4b. The pace was much slower there, and I was able to get to know the children. They were older, and many had dietary problems. Several had coeliac disease.

I was on 4b for my first Christmas at Great Ormond Street. For once we were on duty all day, but no one minded. In any case there was no public transport in London. When we came on duty at 7.30 A.M., the children were already opening their stockings. Each child was given a new set of clothes that day, many of them knitted by the friends of the hospital. All the wards were decorated; anyone with artistic talents was in great demand to paint on the cubicle glass windows. The whole hospital looked like a fairyland. The playroom on each ward was decorated and made into a cosy corner for the staff. The children were bathed and fed and by 10.30 A.M. Everyone was either by the windows or out on the balconies waiting for the arrival of Father Christmas on his sleigh. All the theatre staff were dressed as reindeer, fairies and pantomime characters. Doctors, surgeons, sisters and nurses all took part. Father Christmas then toured the wards, delivering a present to every child. Parents and family were all welcome to visit on Christmas Day. The atmosphere was wonderful.

At lunchtime the consultant of each ward arrived to carve the turkey. The children were all given their Christmas dinner first, and then, while they rested, the doctors joined the nurses for dinner in the playroom. At about three o'clock celebrities, including Tommy Steele, the Two Ronnies, Cliff Richard and many more, arrived to tour the hospital. The children were thrilled to get autographs and talk to their heroes as they toured the wards. After tea a group of nurses with their cloaks on, red side out, came round the wards singing carols.

The chapel at Great Ormond Street was a quiet place where parents, children, doctors, and nurses could find comfort and help at this special time. There was a crib scene to remind us all of the real meaning of Christmas.

After carols, the children gradually started to settle. The mothers and fathers at each side of a bed or cot, each holding a tiny hand. When all was quiet, we nurses settled down to relax and to enjoy the goodies we had received from grateful parents. At 8.00 P.M. the night nurses came on to relieve us. It had been a magical day. Some children were, sadly, too sick to know it had been Christmas Day. Not long after Christmas my set had a two-week holiday.

Veronica and I had booked a trip to go skiing in Norway. It was a wonderful holiday and we got plenty of fresh air and exercise and ate good food.

My next work was in the ear, nose and throat (ENT) theatre. I was there for six weeks but did not really enjoy the experience, although I realised it was a necessary part of my training. The sister who worked in this department was known to be very good at growing delicious tomatoes at her flat. One day after a tonsillectomy operation I found the sister pouring the blood into a large jam jar. When I asked what she was saving it for, she gave me a smile and said it was fertiliser for the famed tomatoes she grew. At first I was horrified but then thought why not? It was no different from the blood and bone fertiliser one bought in plant shops.

Princess Anne came to Great Ormond Street to have her tonsils out. Although I was working in the ENT department at the time, I never actually saw her. Fortunately, there were no complications, and she was soon discharged.

My next three months were spent doing night duty, which I never really enjoyed; it was terribly tiring. We worked for twelve nights and then had four off. The night nurses' home was at Hampstead. We were taken from there to Great Ormond Street each evening by coach. The first night was always a nightmare. The juniors worked between two wards and relieved the seniors for meals. Waiting for us at Hampstead would be a work list from the nurses we were relieving. This list told us the names, ages and diagnoses of the children we were going to look after. On the coach we would all frantically try to memorise these details. Around midnight the night sister would come, and we had to take her round the ward and tell her about each child without referring to the work list.

Another feature of night duty was the "cross book" each nurse in training had. In it were listed all the procedures that a sick children's nurse might have to know, such as stitch removal, bladder washout, intravenous infusion, catheterisation, etc. A trolley or tray had to be correctly laid for each procedure. To obtain a cross for competence we junior nurses would be tested by the night sisters. It was up to us to complete our books before we took our final examinations at the end of three years' training.

One might imagine that a children's hospital would be relatively quiet at night, but not so. Babies need to be fed at frequent intervals, and observations have to be recorded throughout the night. A lot of children are on intravenous infusions, and medicines have to be given. We were busy from 8.00 P.M. until 8.00 A.M. We had a meal break round midnight and an hour off for a rest and tea from about 3.00 A.M. until 4.00 A.M. When we were awakened, how we longed to go on sleeping, especially on the eleventh and twelfth nights of night duty. Somehow we would get going again, make the wards clean and tidy and get the children fed and bathed by the time the day staff relieved us at 8.00 A.M.

I always went home for my four nights off. It was bliss! My mother let me sleep as long as I liked. But it took at least two days to recover and the third and fourth days went much too quickly.

The three months soon passed, and then I did a spell at Tadworth Court, the country department of Great Ormond Street. Tadworth had one ward in the main house and two long pavilions in the spacious grounds. Most of the children at Tadworth were long-term patients—spastics, TB cases, children with congenital orthopaedic deformities, etc. Plaster of paris was used a lot to promote long-term rest or to heal limbs after surgery. Whenever possible, these children had plenty of fresh air and sunshine, their beds were pushed out into the garden and they had schooling and entertainment. I loved the atmosphere at Tadworth; it was much more easygoing, and on the whole the children's prognoses were good. Many had never lived in the country. On the grounds there was a tame donkey, cats and kittens, a dog, rabbits and guinea pigs.

While I was at Tadworth, I bought a scooter because it was a complicated journey to my home in Winchester. I loved my Lambretta. The road via Alton and Petersfield to Winchester was a very pleasant ride, giving me fresh air and a feeling of freedom. The scooter also enabled me to go and visit my elderly great Uncle Willie and Auntie Dolly, who looked after him. They lived at Reigate, which was fairly close to Tadworth. My aunt had worked with Dr Barnados for many years but was now retired so that she was free to be with Uncle Willie, who was in his late eighties. I remember having lots of homemade fudge and other goodies during my visits.

Chapter 3
SECOND AND LAST YEAR AT GOS

When I returned to Great Ormond Street in 1957, I was well into the second year of Registered Sick Children's Nurse (RSCN) training. During the second and third year we spent a six-week period in the nursing school. We wore uniforms and attended lectures from senior consultants, the senior nursing staff and tutors. I found this part of my training fascinating. By this time I had looked after children with many rare diseases and was really interested in knowing more about their diagnosis, symptoms, treatment and nursing care. As a general reference book, we used *Nursing and Diseases of Sick Children* by Alan Moncrieff and A.P. Norman. I still have my copy today and refer to it from time to time. At the end of each six weeks we had to pass exams before we could progress to the next stage of training.

At the start of the second year, the design of our caps changed, so that our seniority would be obvious; it changed again on starting our third year. Towards the end of my second year I worked on the leukaemia ward. In those days the prognosis for this disease was poor. Children were often diagnosed in their local hospitals and then sent to Great Ormond Street for treatment. After a period of chemotherapy they would go home in remission but were nearly always admitted with further symptoms or infections.

I became particularly involved with a little boy called David. He was seven years old and had been in and out of the ward several times. His delightful parents adored him. He had two younger brothers, Nick and Sam. David, who had lost all of his hair because of the chemotherapy, had a mischievous expression, and even when in pain, he was very brave and cooperative.

As a children's nurse, it is inevitable that one sometimes makes a particularly close bond with a child. This happened to me when David was diagnosed as terminally ill. At Great Ormond Street a very sick child would be "specialled". This meant that round the clock, he was never left alone. It was while I was "specialling" David one morning that he held my hand, gave me a faint smile and died. He was the first child I had seen die, and I must admit to feeling scared, angry and devastated. I was scared because I had come to love David and could not understand why such a young child should die. I was devastated because of feeling so inadequate and knowing how distressed his parents would be.

The ward sister asked if it was my first experience with death, and when I told her it was, she proceeded to give me the most important lesson of my children's training, and one for which I shall always be grateful.

Together we washed David all over, removing tubes, stitches and plasters. His bed was made up with clean linen, and his hair was brushed and combed. We then put on a little white gown with frills at the neck and wrists. His hands, holding a tiny bunch of flowers, were gently folded together across his chest. He looked like a peaceful little choir boy. Throughout these ministrations the sister talked to me quietly and explained exactly what she was doing. By the time his parents arrived I felt more confident and less tearful. Young and inexperienced, I did not realise that the ward sister has to break the news to the parents and that it is her responsibility to console them when they arrived. But I had learnt how important it was to spend time with and offer dignified, loving care to a dead child. Thus, when the parents come to see their child before he or she is moved to the mortuary, every care has been taken to ease their grief and pain.

Towards the end of my second year, four of us from my set had a boating holiday on the Thames. We rented a converted barge moored at The Beetle and Wedge, a pub in Moulsford. The owner agreed to take us on a trial run to explain the engine, steering and river code as well as how to navigate a lock. We all listened intently; however, when we actually started upstream on our own towards Abingdon, we experienced all manner of difficulties. The engine stalled midstream, a large, smart cruiser was coming towards us at great speed. There was a lot of shouting and panic, but we managed somehow to wedge ourselves on a muddy bank. Another time we narrowly missed being swept over a weir by the strong current. The funniest and wettest incident occurred when one of our party leant over a bit too far to reach the side of the lock. She made a great splash as she fell from the barge! Fortunately, it was a lovely, hot day, and she was soon clambering back on board.

Each evening we found a quiet mooring within walking distance of a village, where we visited the pub and bought any provisions we needed from the shop. Several times we walked to a farm for fresh milk. One morning we woke to see an inquisitive cow peering into the cabin.

As we approached Abingdon we saw four Royal Air Force officers strolling down the riverside path towards us. They asked us to accompany them to a nearby pub. In those days one was not so wary of strangers, and we happily accepted their invitation. We all had a great time and arranged to meet the following evening for a barbecue on the riverbank.

After our holiday we returned to Great Ormond Street, received our caps and became third-year nurses. I then went to work on the neurosurgical ward. It was a very traumatic ward to work on, but I learned much about the importance of meticulous basic nursing care: the care of the skin, particularly all pressure points, the care of the mouth, the eyes and the airway, the position of all limbs and the importance of passive movements for an unconscious child. A lot of the children were on respirators, so I had to learn how to cope with these machines and watch for any complications or change in these children's conditions. We were taught to talk to unconscious children while we tended them. It was explained to us that no one knew the level of their unconscious state, and although they might not respond to touch, they might be able to hear what was going on round them.

I remember one little girl who had been in a coma for weeks. Katy had been a happy, normal child playing in the park one minute, but the next she was hit hard at the back of her head by a wooden swing. She was rushed to the local hospital and was unconscious on arrival. She had a severe intercranial haematoma and

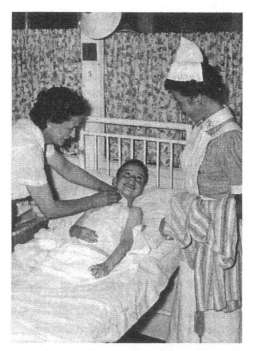

Mary with a patient at Great Ormond Street
Hospital. (Kemsley Picture Service)

needed specialist surgery, so she was transferred to Great Ormond Street and
went straight to theatre. Unfortunately, the pressure had caused brain damage, and
she had not regained consciousness. She could, however, breathe without assistance
and had very slight responses to painful stimuli. The doctors never gave up hope
that in time her damaged brain might recover.

Our job with Katy was to prevent any complications, such as chest infections or
pressure sores. Our careful nursing was rewarded, and Katy did eventually wake
up. She took a long time to convalesce, but with physiotherapy, and our continued
care and the love of her parents, she made a miraculous recovery. I have never
forgotten how she became injured, and ever since then I have always been very
strict with children playing on swings.

A boy we nursed had a horrific injury to his scalp. He had been playing on a
sports field, where the grass was being cut with a large machine. Unfortunately,
the groundsman did not see the child, who fell very close to the knives. A large
flap of the boy's scalp was sliced open. He was rushed to Great Ormond Street by
helicopter. He had lost a lot of blood, and it was feared that he would have a brain
infection. For several days it was touch and go, but he was a strong, healthy child,
and he recovered. The groundsman, full of remorse and guilt, came to the hospital,
and we were able to reassure him and let him see the child playing happily with
toys. This boy was another example of how resilient children can be.

During my third year Princess Alexandra came to spend a few weeks at the hospital. She wanted to learn about normal baby and child care. At the time I was doing my stint in the diet kitchen. Special diet orders came from the wards each morning, and it was our job to prepare them. One morning we arrived to start work as usual, and much to our surprise and excitement, we were told that Princess Alexandra was coming to join us for the day. This tall, cheerful, attractive girl quickly put us all at ease, and we all had a very happy day together.

An unexpected patient admitted to the hospital during my third year, was my niece Judith, aged about eight years; for routine tonsillectomy. I visited her on the ENT ward each morning and evening, and remember feeling so sorry for her, she did not want to eat or drink anything, and looked so miserable. However there were no complications and she quickly recovered and was discharged.

Most of my set celebrated their twenty-first birthdays during their third year of training. Jo's father was on the committee of the All-England Tennis Club, so she was allowed to have her party in the ladies' dressing rooms at Wimbledon. We had a wonderful party. The climax came when we all took off our shoes and did the conga round the centre court.

Towards the middle of my third year, Sheila, one of my boating companions, bought a Lambretta like mine. We decided to spend a ten-day's holiday touring France and Switzerland on my scooter. In the space of ten days we took the ferry to Calais, drove across France into Switzerland via Geneva, then on to Basel and back through France to London. It was a fantastic ten days, and we stayed each night in pensions. I used my school French to book a room each evening.

On our return trip through France, the skies opened, and we got wetter and wetter. We didn't want to stop for fear of missing the ferry. Eventually, we decided to stop at a café to have at least some hot soup. When we walked in, we were dripping puddles on the floor. We must have looked a pathetic sight! The manageress took charge and practically frog-marched us to the ladies' room. In broken English, she told us to take all our clothes off and give them to her. She said she would lock the door so that no one could come in, then she would come back and knock three times and give us hot soup and French bread. We explained that we had a ferry to catch and could not stay long.

We hoped that she would not leave us stranded for too long. Within minutes she had returned as promised with hot, tasty soup and French bread. In less than half an hour she came back with our clothes, which were by now almost dry. We felt completely restored by the time we set off once more for the ferry.

We returned to our last three-month stint of night duty. As third-year nurses, we were each in charge of a ward. To my amazement, I had been assigned to IC, the intensive surgical ward where I had started my training. But this time I would be in charge. I loved that challenging three months. My desire to specialise in intensive care undoubtedly came from that spell of senior night duty on IC.

Many of the babies admitted to IC whilst I was on this ward did survive. Successes were a team achievement, and not the slightest mistake could be made. At night I had to see that every child in my care was properly looked after. Of course the night sisters were always on call for advice, and they made frequent rounds of the wards, but I was the one who had to observe any change in the condition of the ten children in my care.

I did get very tired, both mentally and physically, during that night duty. Twelve nights of constant concentration was a long time, but I gained much confidence and experience. I learnt how to work closely with the surgeons and doctors on the ward and, most importantly, to nurse desperately sick babies.

The three years came to an end, and then I had to pass my final examinations. I gained my RSCN qualification in 1959 and have always felt proud to have trained at Great Ormond Street Hospital for Sick Children.

Chapter 4

GENERAL NURSES' TRAINING AT MIDDLESEX HOSPITAL

During the last few months at Great Ormond Street Hospital we were constantly told that if we wanted to make progress in a nursing career it was imperative to do a two-year training in a general hospital. We would not be able to become sisters of a children's ward unless we had this State Registered Nurse (SRN) qualification. So I decided to apply to the Middlesex Hospital, the famous London teaching hospital, which had a close relationship with Great Ormond Street. I was accepted and began my SRN training almost immediately.

A girl called Mary Simmons, who had been in the set above me at GOS, joined the Middlesex on the same day. We immediately formed a close friendship. She was a small, dark attractive girl and full of fun. We had neighbouring rooms in the John Astor House nurses' home, and when we were on night duty, we shared a double room.

I found the change from nursing children to adults difficult, especially men, because since the age of twelve I had grown up without a father, and my brother was much older than me. I was very shy and unused to close contact with the opposite sex. Having done our children's training, Mary and I joined the three-year general training course at the start of its second year. We therefore missed out on the basics of nursing adults, which I am sure would have made me feel more confident.

My first spell of duty was on the cardiac ward. The consultants were famous, Dr Somerville and Dr Bonham Carter. For rounds, everything had to be immaculate in the ward—beds had to be tidy and in line, and patients had to be clean, sitting up and comfortable. Charts had to be up to date and placed at the foot of each bed. We nurses, too, had to look immaculate, with clean caps and aprons, polished shoes and tidy hair. We stood at attention at the end of the ward in case we were needed.

One consultant did his round at the beginning of the week, the other at the end. At 2.00 P.M. on Monday afternoon a sister entered the ward with Dr Somerville, who was tall, grey haired and very distinguished looking but rather frightening to student nurses. He always wore a buttonhole on the jacket of his dark suit. Friday was the turn of Dr Bonham Carter. He was rather small and untidy looking, but he had a very kind, cheerful expression. Both consultants were followed by their entourage of doctors, registrars, surgeons and medical students. This group stopped for a few minutes at the end of each bed to discuss the case, otherwise there was complete silence while they all toured the ward. There was a sigh of relief when it was all over and the ward could return to its normal routine.

Middlesex student nurses also staffed the Women's Hospital in Soho. We walked in uniform from the night nurses' home, down Oxford Street and into Soho for a stint of night duty. We went in twos and threes, but I never once felt afraid as I walked through the red-light district of Soho; in fact, I used to find it a fascinating experience. Yes, we saw prostitutes standing on the pavements, but they always called out, "Good evening, luv. Have a good night," and we replied, "And you too!" When we came off duty in the morning at 7.30, it all looked quiet and very different.

On a much sadder occasion, I visited my little goddaughter Joanna, who was admitted to the children's ward at St Thomas Hospital with congenital heart disease. She fought so hard for her life, but nothing could be done for her. It was devastating for my great friend, Penny, and her husband, Bob. Penny had been at school with me, and I had been delighted to be asked to be Joanna's godmother.

During our time at the Middlesex Hospital Mary and I had two memorable holidays. The first was a week in Cornwall. By this time I had exchanged my Lambretta for a Mini. Mary had reminded me that the road tax was out of date, so we simply removed it from the windscreen, for I could not afford to renew the licence and be able to go on holiday. We had bed and breakfast in different places each day and enjoyed sunbathing. We had wonderful, clear blue skies and hot sun every day. On the last night, Tig, Mary's fiancé, joined us; the only room we could get had a double bed and a single bed, so Mary and I shared the double, and Tig had the single. We laughed and told many stories that night. The next morning we returned to London, revived, happy and suntanned.

For another holiday Tig took Mary, her sister and me to the Belgian Grand Prix. We went in Tig's car and crossed the channel in a tank-like, one-car air ferry. I was glad when we landed. There were so many people, so much noise and a strong smell of oil and petrol. I had never seen or heard racing cars in action before. Tig was an expert and explained everything to us.

On the way home the exhaust fell off on a fast dual carriageway, and Tig's car made a tractor-like sound. Mary and I had to catch the plane that we had booked, or we would not get back to the Middlesex in time to go on duty, so we stood waving frantically for about ten minutes trying to stop someone and get help. But it was useless. As no one took any notice, we all put on every item of clothing we had, opened all the windows and continued our journey at twenty miles per hour. The cold and the smell of fumes were terrible. When we landed in England, Tig was able to get the exhaust fixed. Mary and I got back just in time to change into uniform and go on duty.

Although we had an incredibly small salary whilst we were training, we did have four weeks' paid holiday each year, usually two weeks in summer and two in winter. Ann, a friend from my set at GOS, joined Mary and me at Middlesex. Ann and I loved skiing so we would go together to Switzerland and France on wonderful two-week Murison Small chalet parties for young skiers. There were usually sixteen to twenty in a chalet, with two girls to cook. The thrill of flying down the steep mountains, the sun, fresh air and the après ski life all added up to fantastic holidays for us. At the end of two years, in 1962, I took my finals and qualified as a state registered nurse.

Chapter 5

MISCELLANEOUS JOBS

After more than five years in London hospitals I was desperate for a change. I wanted to work with normal, healthy children.

I had heard one could find interesting jobs advertised in the *Lady* magazine. It was just luck, or maybe fate, that I bought this one particular copy and took it home. In the back pages I found an advertisement from a titled lady who needed someone to help with her three children during summer holidays at the family's country estate in Berkshire, at their seaside home in Sandwich and at their shooting lodge in the Scottish Highlands.

I telephoned immediately. Lady Samuel answered and asked me to go to London for an interview the next day. Her ladyship explained to me that, as all her children were now at boarding school, her nanny had retired. However, because she entertained a lot, particularly at the shooting lodge, she needed someone to live with them as family and keep an eye on Sarah, who was fourteen, Nicky, who was eleven, and Michael, who was nine.

The next morning, to my surprise, Lady Samuel rang. She wanted me to join the family at their home in Berkshire the following month, when the children were due to break up from school.

Their home turned out to be a very beautiful mansion surrounded by extensive grounds. There was a full staff: a butler, a chauffeur, maids, cleaners, a chef and gardeners.

From the start I was treated as one of the family. Lady Samuel introduced me to Sarah, Nicky, and Michael. At the beginning Sarah was not too easy. Understandably, she felt she was too old to have a stranger keep an eye on her. I realised I would have to win her over and hoped that we could become friends. The boys were very cooperative.

My first task with the three children was to unpack the three trunks, which were full of dirty cloths, school uniforms, towels and bed linen. Then we all set about choosing and packing clothes for the holiday at Sandwich.

There was great excitement on the day we set off in two cars. The parents and Sarah went in the Rolls Royce; the two boys and I went in the second car driven by the chauffeur. The house at Sandwich had five bedrooms and a garden at the back and the front. It was only about half a mile from the sea and the Royal St George Golf Club. The children had spent summer seaside holidays there since they were born. The boys played for hours with their soldiers in the garden sandpit. Sarah had a French exchange girl named Sophie stay for a week. There were not many chores for me to do, so I spent most of the time with the children. We did all the usual seaside things—swimming, shrimping, walking, boating, shell seeking and picnicking.

One day Lady Samuel went off after breakfast to spend the day with friends. I was left in charge of the children and asked to take Sarah to a golf lesson at the club at 11.00 A.M. We all spent an hour or so on the beach, returning to the house in time for Sarah to change. To my horror, I realised that her parents had gone off in the smaller car, and there was only the Rolls Royce for me to use. By this time it was too late to walk, for I had been given strict instructions the night before that Sarah must not miss her golf lesson.

I was quite an experienced driver by this time, but I had certainly never driven a Rolls Royce! I found judging the width of the car very difficult. We had to go down a narrow drive and through some white gates. I was terrified I would damage the bodywork. Thankfully, I got Sarah to the club in time and waited the hour that her lesson lasted. We returned very slowly and arrived back at the house in one piece. I breathed a very big sigh of relief.

After two weeks in Sandwich we returned to Berkshire to prepare for the month in Scotland, the highlight of the children's summer holidays. Our excitement rose as we all arrived at Euston station in London to catch the night sleeper to Scotland.

I had never been to the Highlands of Scotland, and certainly not in a first-class sleeper. The tremendous excitement of the children was infectious. The next morning, when they woke early and looked out of the windows, they shouted and squealed as we passed places they recognised. Eventually, the train pulled into the little Highland station. As we all jumped out of the train, we were met by the staff from the shooting lodge: the chauffeur, the butler and the gamekeeper. It was obvious how fond they were of the children and interested in seeing how much they had grown and changed since their previous visit. I felt a bit like an outsider, but we were soon packed into cars and set off across the moors down a narrow drive about two miles long. The shooting lodge was a long, traditional Highland house with a lawn in front and a burn trickling down the hill at the back.

When we arrived, the children quickly settled into their familiar nursery wing. Sarah and I each had our own room; the boys shared. There was a bathroom and a good-sized room where we could eat, play and sit. In the main part of the house there was a very large dining room and a beautifully furnished and comfortable sitting room. Upstairs their lordships had their own suite of rooms. There were about six guest rooms, each with its own bathroom. At the back of the house was a modern kitchen (a French chef had been employed to cook for the month) and several pantries, laundry and storerooms.

The first week only the family were in residence. The boys spent hours worming for trout in the burn and Sarah loved riding the Highland ponies on the estate. I had to see they had clean clothes to wear, make their beds and supervise their breakfasts and suppers, which were brought to us in the nursery wing. We all had lunch together in the main dining room or had picnics.

During the last three weeks a number of guests arrived for the shooting. Twice a week Lady Samuel invited me to go into the dining room for dinner. I never knew who I was going to sit next to. Everyone wore formal evening dress. The food was absolutely delicious—always five courses, coffee and liqueurs. The conversation was mostly about the days' shooting or the size of trout caught that day.

A typical days' shooting started at 9.30 A.M. I had to make sure the children were dressed sensibly for the weather. We all met in the front drive, where the gamekeepers discussed any final details with his lordship. Sometimes we walked with the guns and I made sure the children all stayed in the line. Sometimes we stood in the butts with the guns waiting for the grouse to fly over us. The lunch picnics were wonderful; all over the hills there were wooden trestle tables which could be erected at lunchtime. At about midday a string of ponies with panniers on their backs led by one or two staff members from the shooting lodge could be seen approaching the picnic spot. Lunch had been prepared by the French chef. The food was marvellous. We had game pies, asparagus rolls, quiches, pate' rolls, smoked salmon sandwiches and beer or wine to drink. The picnic ended with coffee and liqueurs. If it was dry, we sat around on tufts of heather; if it was wet, we tried to find rocks, pieces of wood or waterproof mackintoshes to sit on.

I had the best of both worlds. Not only was I made to feel like one of the family, but I was accepted by all the staff. At the back of the house was a row of cabins, where the students who were employed as beaters lived. On one occasion there was to be a dance in the local village hall, and the beaters had asked me to go with them. I asked Lady Samuel if she minded me going. Not only did she give permission, but she said I could see the chauffeur and borrow one of the smaller cars. She asked me to drive very carefully and not be too late coming home. Mr James, the chauffeur, showed me the car, and we went for a trial run to make sure I was familiar with the gears and lights.

I had a great time at the dance and started home about midnight. I found out later that her ladyship was still up waiting for me to get home safely, but she never heard the car come into the yard. Instead of going straight to bed, I went and had a nightcap with the beaters. It was 2.00 A.M. when I finally crept into the main house. Lady Samuel who, was still up, was by this time frantically worried and her anxiety had made her very angry. When she saw me come in, she told me I could pack my bags and leave in the morning. I had not appreciated how concerned she would be.

I went to bed feeling livid with myself and sorry that I had been so thoughtless. In the morning I went to explain and offer my apologies to her ladyship. To my amazement she forgave me. The incident was never mentioned again.

Some of the guests brought children with them. These children joined us in the nursery for breakfast and supper. They also joined us in entertainment. Occasionally, we would go into the nearest village, where there was a pony-trekking centre. We would go out on the hills all day on mountain ponies with a guide. All the children were good riders, and they loved pony-trekking. These were wonderful days.

Another entertainment was fishing for pike in one of the lochs on the estate. The gamekeeper would prepare the bait, which was made with a bottle that floated and a length of wire with a small fish on the end. The gamekeepers would take me and all the children in long rowing boats across the loch and we dropped about ten baits. The next morning we returned to see what we had caught. Pike are very strong, and it was quite a job to land and kill the fish. Fortunately, no one ever fell in.

Sadly, this very special three months came to an end. We returned on the train to London and on to the family home in Berkshire, where I helped the children get ready for school. I returned home to my mother in Winchester feeling rather deflated. There I discovered that my brother was not well. He was by then out of the army and living with his wife and children in Norwich.

I was worried about him and decided to apply to the Norfolk and Norwich Hospital to see if I could get a staff nurses' post there. I was offered a post on the private block and started working there almost immediately.

My brother was in and out of the hospital at the time. He had three children: Nigel, was six, Sandra two and Edward nearly a year. I loved working so close to them. I saw a lot of the family, especially Nigel, whom I often took for walks. I tried to teach him to swim at the local swimming pool, but without success. I stayed in Norwich nearly nine months, living in a bed-sitter not far from the hospital. During this time I also got to know my godfather, an orthopaedic consultant at the Norfolk and Norwich Hospital.

In the spring of 1963, Lord Samuel's brother asked me to go to Scotland with him and his children, as it was his turn for the shooting lodge. This time there were two girls: Jacqui, who was nearly eighteen, Lavinia, who was fourteen, and their friend Camilla. Again, I had a wonderful month, different, but just as much fun. Later that year I was asked to go with them to their estate on the Spey River in Scotland. I had not experienced salmon fishing before, and I found it fascinating. Both Jacqui and Lavinia were experienced anglers. One day I was lent a rod and told I could go fishing with the butler, he was very keen and never missed an opportunity. After some fifteen minutes, a large salmon rose and took the bait on my line. I was so surprised and inexperienced that instead of playing the fish and letting it take a bit of line, I hung on to it for grim death. The fish took the hook, bait and line and disappeared downstream! I had to confess to his lordship. He laughed and said, "Oh, don't worry. Better luck next time."

When Jacqui turned eighteen, her father gave her a car. Unfortunately, she was allowed to bring it to Scotland. One night I was alone with the girls, and Jacqui decided to go out in her car to visit a friend a few miles away. When she had not returned by 9.00, I was very worried and decided to go out in another car to search for her. I found Jacqui and her car in a ditch. She was terrified but had had the sense to lock all the doors. On a deserted piece of road across the moors she had taken a corner too fast and had shot off the road. She was unhurt but very cold and in shock. We locked her car and returned in mine. Then I had to telephone her father and tell him what had happened. What a considerable responsibility it is looking after other people's children!

On my return to Winchester, I was asked to help two expectant mothers. The first request for help was from my old school friend Penny. Her husband, Bob, was stationed in the army in Germany. The second came from Julie, another school friend who lived in Sussex and was expecting her third child. The problem was that Julie's baby was due two weeks before Penny's. How would I manage to help both of them?

I arrived in Sussex a few days early to look after Amanda, aged three, and Nicholas, aged eighteen months, whilst Julie was in the hospital. Several days later, when the baby had still not arrived, we become more worried, for I was booked to fly to Penny's in a week's time. Julie and I had heard that castor oil could help to start labour, so we set off for the nearest chemist. The shop was closed, but Julie was determined. She knocked on the door, and the village pharmacist obligingly gave us medicine. We went home, and Julie took the dose of castor oil. Julie started labour pains that evening, and she was admitted to hospital. Little Annabelle was delivered before midnight.

Julie came home forty-eight hours later; Annabelle was a beautiful, healthy baby. She slept in my room for the first four nights, and I gave her the night feeds in order to give Julie a good rest. During the day Julie and I looked after the three children together. I had to leave a week later and catch my flight to Germany.

I was met at the airport by Bob, Penny's husband, and their son, Tim, who was five that day. Penny had been admitted to the hospital early, and her normal, healthy baby had arrived that morning. Since Tim had some friends coming to his birthday tea party and there was no cake, Tim asked if I would please make a train cake. I was not a very experienced cook, but somehow I managed to make a sponge train with trucks, which we filled with Smarties. Tim and his friends were thrilled with it, which was all that mattered. Saying that she had a Great Ormond Street nurse to look after them, Penny managed to get herself and her baby, Antonia, discharged within twenty-four hours. Once again I had a tiny newborn baby sharing my bedroom.

I was now beginning to feel I should go back to nursing sick children. I wanted to specialise in the cardiac field. Since my brother had moved to Southampton, I applied to the Southampton Chest Hospital and was given a staff nurse's post on the children's postoperative cardiac ward. The experience was invaluable, and I remained there for a year. It was exciting work, as the cardiac consultant surgeon was pioneering new paediatric open-heart surgery. There was a lot of emotional strain as these children often had only a fifty-fifty chance of survival. On the other hand, these children would have died in a year or so without surgery.

Chapter 6
MY FIRST FOUR TRIPS WORKING ON THE *CANBERRA*

While working at the Southampton Chest Hospital, I had a bed-sitter in a house on the edge of New Forest. My journeys to and from work took me past the docks, and I became increasingly aware of where the large passenger liners were frequently berthed. Travelling became more and more tempting.

During my training at Great Ormond Street Hospital word had gone round that the P & O shipping line sometimes employed GOS nurses as children's hostesses; but applicants had to be at least twenty-five, which I wasn't when I was at GOS. I was twenty-seven now, so I decided to write to the P & O head office and was sent application forms. There were a lot of detailed questions to be answered along with request for three references. I was pleasantly surprised when some two weeks later I was asked to go to the P & O head office in London.

This first interview was a fairly simple affair, just myself and a middle-aged personnel manager, but it was much more crucial than I at the time realised. Only very few applicants were ever given a second interview. However, to my amazement I was asked to go to London again for another interview. This time it was terrifying. Having smartened myself up, I arrived at the P & O office in Trafalgar Square and was asked to wait a few minutes. I was very nervous by the time a large double door was opened and I was ushered into a spacious board room. About ten men and one woman were sitting round a long mahogany table.

I was then put through an intensive half-hour interview. At one stage I felt there were doubts about my ability to cope with the job, but one man seemed particularly impressed with my Sherbourne School reference and made a point of saying how much he admired the headmistress. Then out of the blue one of the interviewers asked me how I would cope if I was sent aboard the *Canberra* and had to look after 400 children. How could I answer that question? I had no teacher training and no experience sailing on a liner or coping with large numbers of children. I do not remember what I said, but soon after I was asked this question I was dismissed and told that they would write me. It would have been lovely to have been a fly on the wall after I left the room. I was accepted and asked to join the SS *Canberra* in eight weeks' time when she was due to sail. A list of appropriate clothes to wear when I was on duty was enclosed—navy blue in cold weather conditions and white in hot climates. Also, a separate list of measurements had to be completed and returned immediately, so that my sea-green cocktail dress uniform could be made.

It was all too good to be true. The eight weeks passed quickly, and before I knew it I was on my way to Southampton. My mother and sister came to see me off to Australia!

As we approached the docks, we could see this fantastic white ship. She seemed so high—deck upon deck upon deck. I could see the bridge and the radar just above. There were gangways fore and aft, with a Goanese steward standing at the top of each. I did not know what to do or where to go. I don't think I have never felt so helpless or unsure of myself. I had instructions to report to the purser's office at 11.00 A.M. The passengers were not due to board until midafternoon. I was to be the tourist-class children's hostess.

My boss was sitting across his desk from me. He was small, efficient and looked very smart in his uniform. "Miss Gedge, you have four hundred and fifty children in your care onboard for this trip to Australia." How could I possibly cope with that number of children? Almost as an afterthought, he added, "Don't worry too much. Miss Gothard will put you straight. She has been the tourist-class children's hostess and has moved up to first class. She has coped well and will give you lots of tips. Nearly all the children in your care will be from large families emigrating to Australia. Some of them will be very wild. You will have two Australian girls who are working their way home to give you a hand in the older children's playroom. All I ask is that you keep the children amused so that they do not annoy the passengers in the public lounges. Please be at children's breakfast promptly at seven-thirty each morning so that we can have a chat about any problems." With this he dismissed me.

I walked out in a daze. My mother and sister were waiting outside the office. "I can't possibly cope. There will be four hundred and fifty children onboard in tourist-class this voyage." My mother, in her usual encouraging and confident way, said, "Of course, you can. Come on. Ask where your cabin is."

In the purser's office an attractive dark-haired girl named Mary Baxter offered to show me my cabin on the sun deck. There was accommodation for about a dozen female officers on this deck. I had a fantastic cabin with a window looking out over the sun deck and a first-class swimming pool below. My mother realised how nervous I was and almost immediately she said, "You'll be all right now. We had better get off the ship, or we will be stowaways." After a big hug they left.

So there I was, knowing no one onboard, totally untrained, in a beautiful cabin on the first-class sun deck of the P & O flagship SS *Canberra*. I started to unpack, still in a daze. After only a few minutes there was a knock on my door, and Liz Gothard came in.

Within seconds I knew I'd like Liz. She had been tourist-class children's hostess for the previous year. She knew it all—the good parts, the pitfalls, the routine, what to do and where to go. She was a qualified infant teacher and was also very artistically and musically talented.

But now the passengers were starting to come onboard. The purser had given me a passenger list; on it were the names of the children travelling. My first job as tourist-class children's hostess was to find out the names of all children who would have birthdays while we were at sea so that there would be a birthday cake on the table at children's tea. My next duty was to visit all the cabins where there was a child under one year to ask if tins of baby food or milk were required. I soon found out that there were often six or more children in most of these emigrating families; one family had four sets of twins from the age of two to ten years.

Liz then showed me round the tourist nursery and introduced me to my two stewardesses. These two competent ladies were easy-going and very capable. They had been on the *Canberra* since her maiden voyage three years earlier. They looked after all the under-fives for me. The nursery was wonderfully equipped. There was a Wendy house, a roundabout, a rocking horse, climbing blocks, a tunnel and a mini-bridge with a helm and ship's compass. Because there were so many children onboard for the voyages to Australia, part of the public area next to the nursery called the Island Room was partioned off for the older children's use. I entertained children between the ages of five and twelve in this room. Really, my job was to make the playroom so enjoyable that the children would want to go there.

A typical day for me began with children's breakfast at 7.30. All children under the age of twelve had a special children's menu and their own meal time, which was an hour before the adult first sitting. I had to be in the tourist dining room promptly at 7.30. My boss, the purser, was strict about this. Unfortunately, it was the duty I found hardest, especially if there had been a good party the night before; however much I tried he always got there before me. Then there was a mad dash to get the morning's activities ready. The P & O Company provided everything to keep children amused: paints, felt pens and crayons, paper of all kinds, scissors, glue, plastic modelling kits, Play-Doh, games for all ages and jigsaw puzzles.

Sometimes by 9.00, when I had to open the door to the over-fives, there could be over two hundred children in a queue waiting to come in. Liz advised me to start the mornings with one creative activity, for instance, to suggest that everyone cut out, paint or colour a fish of their own design. My first problem was to make myself heard. Liz suggested I should tell everyone as they entered the playroom to go and sit on the three large mats with their hands over their mouth. This worked like magic! When the children were all quietly seated, I showed them the equipment I had already laid out on the tables. I then explained that we were going to make a very large aquarium on the glass wall dividing our playroom from the rest of the Island Room.

I was always amazed at the talent we had onboard. But, as with all groups of children, there were the troublemakers. Some of the older boys were very rough, and I had to make sure from the start they knew I was boss in the playroom. It only took one or two days for these children to settle, and amazingly they were the ones who were the most helpful once they realised the projects weren't like schoolwork and that there was such a wide variety of activities. Fights were usually between boys in one family. I had one family of five boys who came regularly to my playroom. I became very attached to some of the children in my care during their voyage to Australia.

The first two hours were important, as the children's parents were having breakfast. If the children were not in the playroom with me, they were most likely playing havoc around the ship. Once, a boy of eleven broke the glass and pressed the "man overboard" alarm. (At this signal the engines of the *Canberra* would stop immediately, and the ship would turn in a vast circle. All available crew and officers then would have to scan the sea for a man overboard. This operation would cost the P & O Company an enormous amount of money, so they were not very pleased when it was a false alarm.) The worst part was that even after a plea by the captain over the ship's tannoy for information about who set off the alarm, no one came forward. The ship had circled three times, and as no one had been spotted in the sea, the search was called off and the *Canberra* continued on her voyage.

All the passengers and staff onboard were told to report to the purser's office in case they discovered anyone missing. In the meantime, I was asked to report to the purser. He was very angry, as it was looking more and more likely that one of the tourist children had pressed the alarm and was too afraid to own up. I visited the cabins where I thought the most likely culprit might be and spoke to countless children and parents.

There was a very uneasy atmosphere on the ship for a few hours while the roll call was completed. To the crew's relief, everyone was accounted for, and this was announced over the ship's tannoy. I cannot remember how we finally discovered that the culprit was an eleven-year-old boy who was emigrating with his family to Australia.

Later in the mornings the number in my playroom would thin out. Different activities were put on each table. There was always a crowd round the Lego table, but other favourites were the sewing table and the modelling table. At this stage I could talk to individual children and get to know their names.

Children's lunch was at midday, and after I had seen they were settled at the tables, I was off duty until 2.00 P.M. Since the nursery and my playroom opened again at 1.00—so the children could play whilst their parents had their lunch—one of my stewardesses manned the room until I returned. If the weather was cold, a lot of children spent the afternoon in the playroom. When the sea was rough and the ship was rolling, many of the children felt seasick. I learnt by experience to tell the children to go straight to the buckets, which I had placed at each end of the playroom. If they came to tell me they felt sick, it was usually too late. I explained to the

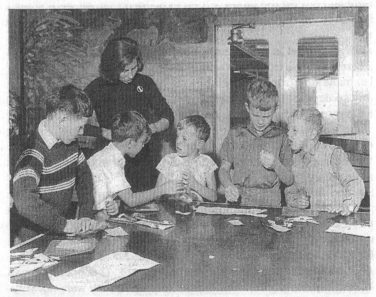

Making plastic aeroplanes in the playroom under my supervision. (Willoughby Gullachsen, Photographic Illustrator)

children that it is quite normal for people to be sick in rough weather. To my horror I had to visit the bucket several times myself the first trip, but luckily, I soon acquired sealegs.

At about four-thirty in the afternoon we would start a mammoth clearing up; fortunately, a steward was sent to help each day. The mess of snips of paper, pieces of wool and cotton and all sorts of other bits and pieces was amazing. Trying to clear up during the day was useless, because within half an hour it was just as bad again. Some of the girls, however, became regular volunteers, and we tried to reward them with a special treat. A visit to the first-class dining room just to have a peep at the cold buffet was popular, as was the loan of a popular game so they could play in the evening when the playroom was closed.

As we sailed into warmer climates I was able to spend more time in the afternoons manning the children's swimming pool. I loved this part of my job on the Canberra. I always wore a bathing costume in case I had to jump in the pool to help a child in difficulty. The pool was not deep, but sometimes it was so crowded that I had to watch the children very carefully, indeed. Most days I gave swimming lessons to those children who were keen to learn. During my first trip to Australia I taught about twenty children to swim. If we felt a child had really learnt to swim during the voyage, the captain would sign a certificate for him or her.

Liz gave me all sorts of suggestions on how to keep the children amused. We had art exhibitions, and the children were invited to bring parents to see the paintings. I always thought the four- to six-year-olds produced the best pictures, for they were so bold and imaginative. Sometimes we would make masks or collages or sew purses; this, surprisingly, was a favourite with the boys as well as the girls.

During the voyage there were all kinds of entertainment laid on for the children. Twice a week I escorted all the children in my playroom to the ship's cinema to see a wonderful selection of cartoons and films. One morning a week I was allowed the use of the live band onboard for musical games. These were very popular sessions, and the band helped me a lot; when we played the zoo game, the band played suitable music for elephants, and if I told the children to be snakes, the band changed the music accordingly. I quickly learned to use a microphone, as it was the only way I could possibly organise and control so many children in one room.

After the first day or so aboard the ship I was feeling very seasick, and I had almost lost my voice from shouting so much to the children in the playroom. When we reached Naples, our first port of call, I was exhausted, Liz was the children's hostess on port duty, so I retired to my bunk for a much needed long sleep. But by the time we sailed again I had got my second wind. The weather was starting to improve, the children were more settled to the routine at sea, my voice returned, and I started to enjoy life again.

The first officer had come to my cabin on our first night at sea to welcome me to the Canberra. He obviously expected me to offer him a drink. I was so green and inexperienced that I had no alcohol in my cabin. Understanding my predicament, he told me that I should give the cabin steward a list of what I needed and suggested a bottle of gin and whisky, some tonics, sodas and cigarettes. He said he would return the following night. My Goanese steward was very helpful, and when I returned from the playroom the next day, the cabinet was full, and an icebox and glasses were ready for use. True to his word, the first officer arrived that evening with the staff captain. We each had a large gin and tonic in my cabin, and they provided me with a lot of useful information.

The captain of the *Canberra*, the senior ship of the P & O fleet, was Commodore Dunkley. During the first few days of each voyage, he hosted a cocktail party in his quarters for specially invited guests. Children's hostesses were not officially on duty after children's tea, but Liz and I were nearly always invited to act as hostesses at these parties. We wore our cocktail dress uniforms, which were really very attractive. The adult social hostesses, the captain's secretary and some of the female pursers were also invited.

On our way to Sydney we called at Alexandria, Port Said, Colombo, Fremantle and Melbourne. We were at sea for three and half weeks. A variety of special entertainments was laid on for the children. One was a visit to the bridge. In the playroom I lined up all those children who were interested in the visit and gave them a short talk on how they must behave sensibly; I then led the crocodile along the deck and up to the bridge. Once on the bridge, the deck officers looked after them, answered questions and showed the children various pieces of equipment. Photographs were taken of the children wearing the officers' uniform hats. These pictures were displayed the next day outside the ship's shop for parents to purchase.

Another afternoon there was the traditional fancy dress parade and party. Liz and I hated these, and eventually we managed to get the staff captain to give permission for us to have theme parties instead. We did not like the competitive fancy dress parades, for we wanted a party that would involve all the children. So we had pirate parties, Indian parties and island parties. In fact, these parties made a lot more work for Liz and I, because we decorated the Island Room to be suitable for each theme. The children made the essential parts of their costumes the day before the party in the playroom, and we gave them any assistance they needed. Indian headdresses were cut out, painted and fixed together, garlands of flowers were made out of crepe paper, and grass skirts were cut out of brown wastepaper bags. We found all the children wanted to join in. It was amazing how realistic the costumes looked. Most children wore their bathing suits as base, and Liz and I helped with makeup, if necessary, for there were face paints in our playroom stock. There were no prizes at these theme parties, just a parade to live band music in front of the captain and some of his deck officers. This was a very popular entertainment for all the tourist passengers onboard. The Island Room was always filled to capacity. The party was followed by a special tea in the dining room for all the children, and a present from the P & O Company was given to each child.

On my first voyage I was responsible for choosing and wrapping 450 toys. There was a huge toy stockroom in the bowels of the ship. Once I made a list of children in each group, I visited this room and chose what I wanted. (On the ship's return to Southampton I had to fill out an order to replace these toys!) Then there was the business of wrapping and naming each present. Liz and I had a marvellous idea. Parties amongst the officers onboard were called "pour outs". So we held "wrapping pour outs". Offices invited were asked to wrap at least ten presents when they came. We had some wonderful parties, and once the officers got going with the wrapping the job was soon done. While these presents were being given out to the children, I was always afraid I had forgotten someone. Although most of the families onboard were travelling on emigration fares that cost ten pounds, the parents would complain bitterly if any of their children did get forgotten; some parents even had the audacity to say their child didn't like their present and asked to have it changed!

One of the main attractions for all the tourist passengers was the "crossing-the-line" ceremony. Several of the officers dressed up as King Neptune and his court. All the children assembled round the swimming pool at the aft end of the ship. Clad in their swimming gear, they sat expectantly in the glorious sunshine. A throne and chairs were put in position, and in front of these was a three-foot-deep square paddling pool. In my white dress uniform, I controlled the children while we all waited for the ceremony to begin. At the appointed time, the ship's bell rang out, after which King Neptune and his followers arrived and took their seats. It was then decreed that Miss Gedge, the tourist-children's hostess, must be found, caught and punished. Of course, this caused uproar amongst the children. In the meantime the deck stewards had hidden me in a corner behind some bags. There was a pretend search, then I was captured and taken to kneel in front of King Neptune. My punishment, much to the delight of the children, was to have sausages, ice cream and all sorts of mess poured out of buckets over my head. I had not realised I would have to play the part of ship's clown when I became tourist-children's hostess! Then I was dipped in the pool. By this time I knew most of the officers who were dressed up; they were a good bunch, and the whole thing was great fun. After each ceremony I did, however, insist on having a free session with the ship's hairdresser. After I had been dipped, the children took it in turn to kneel before King Neptune, and then they, too, were dipped in the pool. The next day they each received a crossing-the-line certificate signed by the captain.

When the weather was good, with the quartermaster's help I organised children's sports on deck. These were very popular. We had all the usual team races: egg and spoon races, sack races, obstacle races, etc. The winners were given tubes of Smarties for prizes. (Liz and I have often wondered if any stray Smarties were found when the *Canberra* was used in the Falkland Islands War some years later.)

When the *Canberra* was in port, most of the passengers went ashore to explore or go shopping. Either the tourist- or first-class nursery stayed open for emergencies. This meant Liz and I could take turns going ashore. Because I had missed Naples, Liz insisted that I went ashore when we reached Alexandria, saying that it was my first trip and that she had done it all before. So I did.

By the time we reached Sydney I realised that the clothes I had bought to wear when I was on duty were much too formal. I had to get some which were a bit more feminine and fashionable. We all had three days off in Sydney, so Liz took me to a wonderful shop where you chose a pattern and material, the seamstress measured you, and the garment you had ordered would be ready for collection next day.

The return to Southampton was very different. There were only about eighty children onboard, nearly all from successful emigrant families who had saved up to go back to England to see their grandparents and family. The send-off for the *Canberra* from Sydney was wonderful. Thousands of streamers of all colours were thrown from the ship to the quay. A band played cheerful music as the huge ship edged her way towards the Sydney Harbour Bridge, then turned and went full steam ahead past the partly built Sydney Opera House. We were followed by a stream of little boats out to sea.

Now my life was not nearly so hectic. The children seemed much more appreciative and better behaved. Since we had set sail four days before Christmas, the staff captain asked me to have a nativity play produced by the children for the tourist-class passengers. Liz was a fantastic help, and so were some of the mothers. For the shepherds we used sheets from the bunks and fathers' dressing gown cords, and one of the mothers had a suitable dress for Mary. Wings for the angels were made out of crepe paper, and we borrowed a real baby for Jesus. We held hasty carol practices, but as usual the children came up trumps on the afternoon of the play, and their little production was much appreciated.

When we reached Southampton I had a week off at home, and then I was off to Australia with another crowd of emigrating families. In all, I worked four emigrating trips to Australia. There were at least four hundred children onboard each trip. These were the last emigrants to go to Australia by sea on the *Canberra*.

Chapter 7
CANBERRA CRUISES

Having survived my first four emigrating voyages to Australia, I felt my apprenticeship was over. The *Canberra* was now scheduled to spend six two-weeks cruises in the Mediterranean. We sailed from Southampton on 12 June 1965 for the first cruise. The elegant white hull and two yellow funnels aft made the *Canberra* quickly recognisable; during cruises she was decked overall with colourful bunting. It was a beautiful summer evening as we slipped past the Isle of Wight and out to sea. Liz, three of the officers and I stood on the upper deck watching the sun go down as the *Canberra* surged through the waves on her way to Cannes, our first port of call.

My basic duties were much the same: children's meals, organise parties, take the children on visits to the bridge and supervise the swimming pool for "children-only" sessions in the afternoons. I still had two stewardesses in the nursery; they worked from 9.00 A.M. until 5.00 P.M. There were only about eighty children onboard, most of them under five. As the older children were on holiday with their parents and the weather was so good, most of the children spent their time swimming or playing deck games. I felt almost redundant. Now was my chance to relax a bit, see the world and have a good time.

Not long after lunch, while sailing from Cannes to Alexandria, the staff captain broadcast a message over the ship's loudspeaker system telling the passengers that a crew member of a French ship in our vicinity had been badly burnt. The *Canberra* was going to alter course in order to transfer the seaman for treatment in our well-equipped hospital. A few hours later we came alongside the French ship and picked up the casualty. The *Canberra's* accident boat and team were used, and the whole operation—a mercy call—was most efficiently and carefully carried out. The staff captain kept the passengers informed. At Alexandria the victim was transferred to a burns unit ashore. We were later told that he made a good recovery and was flown home to France.

In Alexandria I had the afternoon off and went ashore with two of the adult hostesses, Lionel and Penny. We took a taxi along the coast for about half an hour to the old palace that once belonged to King Farouk. In the beautiful grounds were many unusual flowering trees and shrubs and colourful flower beds.

We found a lovely stretch of clean sand, with tables and chairs under large, colourful umbrellas. At the end of a lazy afternoon of swimming and basking in the sun, when it was cooler, we hired the same taxi and did some sightseeing around Alexandria.

We passed an enormous sports centre, where one could play more or less any game, and there was a vast swimming pool. As we returned to the harbour, I realised how busy it was. On one side the disastrous Suez invasion was still remembered; for this reason the British were not popular in Alexandria, and the authorities made difficulties over landing passes and other formalities. The next day a group of us went to the sports centre, and we swam in and sunbathed by the Olympic-sized swimming pool. Four of us discovered we could hire tennis racquets, balls and a court with ball boys, all for five shillings, so we played a few sets of tennis.

The *Canberra* sailed in the evening and headed for Palma on the island of Majorca. This place brought back happy memories of a two-week holiday that I had shared with my mother at Puerto Soller, a fishing village over the mountains from Palma.

Palma has a beautiful, wide harbour surrounded by a large sailing marina and many beaches. When I visited Palma on the *Canberra* in 1965 it was becoming a popular tourist attraction, and many new hotels were being built; but it was not spoilt with block upon block of hotels and apartments as it is today. On the horizon we could see the magnificent cathedral.

When we arrived at Palma, the weather was perfect; a party of some twenty officers, male and female, went off in one of the lifeboats to a nearby island for the day. Having served with the P & O Company for many years, many of the officers were experienced seamen, so we always felt safe on these trips. We took picnic baskets of food with us, and the men brought large containers of iced Bacardi and orange juice, which was deliciously refreshing—and deceptively alcoholic!

On my second cruise, our first stop was Las Palmas in the Canary Islands. We anchored in the harbour and went ashore to explore this uninviting place, which had a lot of volcanic-type mountains in the centre. Along the coast of the island there were blocks of modern flats and hotels. While waiting to go ashore, an enormous battleship came into the harbour; the crew looked very smart in their uniforms as they lined the decks.

At Madeira we anchored offshore, and I was lucky enough to get a spare seat on a passenger trip ashore. My first impressions were of a fertile island with the most wonderful flowers and shrubs growing round the houses and in window boxes. Everything was bright and colourful in the sunshine. As our coach drove along narrow, crowded streets, we passed splendid old buildings, the cathedral and a most beautiful flower market. The road climbed higher and higher. On the way we passed local women in their gardens at work on the famous embroidery. At last we arrived at the top of the famous toboggan run. We could see the *Canberra* below, which looked more like a toy ship instead of an enormous liner. Four of us then sat in a wooden toboggan, which was steered by two men in national costume, and we hurtled down the narrow, twisty, cobbled street to the harbour.

I have returned to Madeira since, and I still love it. I will always remember my first sight of the island from the deck of the *Canberra*, for it was just as beautiful when we sailed at sunset on our way to Palamos, then back to Southampton. The third cruise began on a beautiful summer evening in July. We arrived at Naples four days later. This time, as it was a cruise visit, we had the whole day and evening off. I joined a passenger tour going to Pompeii. We walked four miles with a guide in the scorching sun and got very hot and tired. It was relief to return to my air-conditioned cabin for a cool shower.

In the evening four of us found an excellent pizza bar; it was the first time I had seen pizzas made in front of us on a floured board. I was amazed at the chef's speed and dexterity as he tossed the dough from one hand to the other. Eventually, when he had each pizza shaped to perfection and covered it with our chosen topping, he placed it on a square board attached to a long pole. This was then pushed deep into a very hot oven. The chef checked each pizza at regular intervals until it was cooked to his satisfaction. These pizzas, eaten with ice-cold beer or local wine, made a delicious meal. Whenever I went ashore, I was always worried that I would return late and miss the *Canberra's* departure. In Naples two of the crew did just that! They had hired scooters for the day, but somehow they lost their way and went much farther than they had intended. One of the scooters broke down to boot. They arrived back to see the *Canberra* just sailing out of the harbour. Fortunately, someone with a powerful speedboat brought them out to the *Canberra*. They were able to come aboard when the pilot left the bridge and before the side gangway was removed. They were very lucky and received only a severe reprimand.

We next headed for Greece. This would be my first visit to Athens, but when we went ashore, it was too hot to do much exploring. A group of us spent most of the afternoon at a little café in the shade on the seafront eating delicious locally caught sardines and drinking ouzo. We were surrounded by Greeks. Some drank, whilst others played cards. It was a peaceful way to spend a few hours off the ship. Once back onboard we set off for Portugal. We berthed at Lisbon, and again I was able to go ashore. We took a little train along the coast to the fishing port of Estoril. There we wandered round a large market with an amazing assortment of fish laid in ice on slabs of marble.

Liz, who had by this time become a close friend of mine, was now courting her future husband, a senior deck officer. I was very friendly with one of the engineer officers. Although Liz and I continued as first- and tourist-class children's hostesses, with so few children onboard we were always free at midday to go to drink parties, and these were plentiful. The playroom telephone was kept busy with invitations for us to attend passenger and officer pour outs. After children's tea we were off duty and sometimes helped with adult entertainment, such as horse-race meetings or quizzes. Liz and I both loved dancing. Officers were encouraged to mix with the passengers in the evenings, and live bands were always playing in the tourist- and first-class ballrooms.

Liz started a crew choir called the Glee Club. This was very popular with the crew, who were much more confined to their own living quarters than we officers were. From time to time Liz and the Glee Club put on a concert for the passengers.

While we were sailing from Lisbon back to Southampton, I joined Liz's choir for my first concert. We sang Gilbert and Sullivan and other well known songs from musicals and led community singing.

By my fourth cruise I was very brown and feeling extremely fit. There were no surprises this time, ports of call being Gibraltar, Alexandria and Palma. There were about one hundred children onboard, slightly more than on the previous cruises because the schools had broken up for the summer holidays.

I started to give swimming lessons again, as I had done on the emigrating trips to Australia. The tourist swimming pool depth of water was lowered to about three feet for the "children-only" sessions in the afternoons. The children who wished to learn came for the first half hour, and they were amazingly keen. The P & O Company provided rings and armbands for those who wished to borrow them. I organised swimming races for the older children, they particularly enjoyed the various obstacle races which we invented.

My fifth cruise in August 1965 provided me with the opportunity to get a glimpse of Turkey. I remember most the wonderful spires rising over the city, the tremendous roar of traffic and the bustle of people.

My final cruise left Southampton at the end of the school holidays, so there were very few children onboard. In a way there was sadness, as Liz had decided to return to teaching. I think she wanted to see how she would feel in life ashore away from the deck officer of who she had become so fond, for if she did marry a merchant seaman, she would have to get used to months of separation. Liz and I had become good friends, and I knew that I would miss her greatly. However, we made the most of our last cruise together and had a wonderful time visiting two of our favourite places, Lisbon and Madeira.

My next big adventure was about to begin. I had signed on for the *Canberra's* next three-month voyage, still as children's hostess in the tourist-class. A most experienced children's hostess would transfer from another ship to replace Liz in first class.

Chapter 8
MY FIRST LONG CANBERRA VOYAGE

I returned to the *Canberra* without Liz, my best girlfriend and ally onboard. Ian, who had given me such wonderful times both on the ship and ashore, had been transferred to another P & O liner. Moreover, I had changed. I was mature and confident, able to deal with any situation and converse with anyone. Miss Gedge, the tourist-children's hostess, was now an established member of the *Canberra* crew.

Commodore Dunkley ran a very tight ship. He expected a lot from all his officers and the crew, and because we liked and respected him, we did our best. The staff captain was in charge of entertainment. During my time with P & O, I worked with two staff captains, and each one was approachable and helpful. Once a week we would meet to discuss the week's plans for entertaining the children. On the whole, we did not socialise with the senior officers unless we were formally invited to their passenger cocktail parties when we acted as hostesses. But on one occasion I was invited to join the commodore's party going ashore in Panama City. A friend of his was giving a dinner at his house. The evening was wonderful, and I saw a very relaxed and amusing side of the captain.

Both the Commodore and the staff captains gave me much support for my children's parties. I made them feathered headdresses to wear as Red Indian chiefs, garlands of paper flowers for island parties and black patches and hats for pirate parties. The commodore and staff captains were very sporting and joined in the fun while all the delighted children paraded before them in their costumes.

The rest of the officers were our friends and colleagues. Some eight girls were hostesses, and others worked in the purser's office. Then there were the nursing sisters. I kept my cabin with a window looking out over the first-class swimming pool all the time I was on the *Canberra*. A wonderful Goanese steward looked after us. He seemed to sense when rough weather was expected and always managed to secure all of our breakable items in the cabins before any damage was done. He was a very cheerful and friendly but respectful steward, and he loved to tell us about his wife and children at home in Goa.

My immediate boss, the purser, was continually sending for me, sometimes at very awkward moments, to complain about something I had omitted to do or something I had done which he felt was wrong. Perhaps it was just to keep me on my toes and remind me he was in charge. However, he cannot have thought too badly of me, as he gave me a very good report at the end of each voyage. Towards the end of my time at sea we became good friends.

When I reported to him in September 1965 for the long voyage, he told me there were 100 children in tourist class and that I could use one side of the Island Room (next to the playroom) to entertain the older children, as I had done for the emigration runs to Australia.

Before sailing from Southampton, we always had a boat drill. Every member of the ship's company had his or her own station on deck. When the alarm sounded, quickly and quietly we made our way to the correct station. The whole ship's company was then inspected by the captain and senior officers, and the emergency equipment and lifeboats were checked. I became increasingly interested in ship safety and enrolled for lifeboat drill classes. There was much to learn, and when I passed the oral and practical examination in Vancouver, I was awarded a lifeboatman certificate of efficiency. I now knew how to take a lifeboat from the upper decks to the sea and get it away from the ship in an emergency.

In the few hours before the passengers embarked, I was delighted to find that several families would be returning to Sydney via America. This meant I would have a good nucleus of children onboard who knew me and the routine at sea.

This was to be my first visit to America. We were due to sail via Port Everglades in Florida to the Bahamas and through the Panama Canal to Acapulco, Los Angeles, San Francisco, up the coast to Vancouver and then to Honolulu, Auckland and Sydney.

As I stood below the bridge and we glided out of Southampton Water, I trained my binoculars on the end of the pier and saw my mother, sister and Anthony, my nephew, eagerly waving. It was a great send-off. I felt quite emotional, knowing that I would not see them for about three months. When I could no longer see them, I returned to my cabin and found a beautiful bouquet of flowers my mother had sent. Fresh flowers, green grass and villages with their little churches and pubs were things I missed terribly whilst I was at sea.

One of my playroom stewardesses was new. Unluckily for her, for the first two days we had the roughest seas that I could remember since I had joined the *Canberra*. Even Commodore Dunkley and the senior deck officers said it was unusually rough. However, the bad weather soon passed, and on the third morning we awoke to glorious sunshine and clear blue skies.

Was it my father's influence and memories of lively children's services at his church in Guilford that made me want to organise a service for the children on Sundays when we were at sea? Among the passengers was a young clergyman with his wife and baby; they were on their way to New Zealand. The clergyman was delighted to help arrange services on deck. Most of the children came and joined in singing hymns and choruses accompanied by a pianist, another volunteer from the tourist passengers. We chose older boys and girls to read from the Bible or say prayers. The service was short, but many parents were grateful.

"A Treasure Island" was chosen as the theme for the dressing-up party. Boys were to come as pirates and girls as hula-hula girls. Large numbers of enthusiastic children came to the playroom each morning to cut and stick and sew. About ten of the oldest children helped me to decorate the Island Room with palm trees, crepe paper flowers and garlands on the morning of the party. Two deck officers saw all these preparations going on and offered to dress up and bring in the treasure chest containing the presents. As the one-legged Long John Silver, one young officer had to bend his leg, strap it to his thigh and then fix a wooden leg to his doubled-up knee. It was nearly a disaster. The blood almost stopped circulating in his strapped leg and was terribly painful by the end of the party.

We passed through the Panama Canal in daylight. I lined all the older children up along the deck outside the Island Room and gave each child a drawing book and pencils. The idea was for them to draw anything interesting that they saw so that they had a homemade memento to keep. Some of the results were fascinating.

We passed through a thick jungle with tall palm trees and cactus-type plants. In between the four huge locks there were long stretches of water, similar to lakes. All morning it was very hot and steamy. By lunchtime we were glad to be in the air-conditioned dining room. All afternoon we continued through the canal. The children had become bored with the jungle scenery by this time, so I organised party games in the air-conditioned Island Room.

During the day two Americans had done a running commentary of interest over the ship's broadcast system. Ann, my nursing sister friend, and I were invited to go ashore with them when we reached the end of the canal. They drove us up a steep hill, then we walked through fairly long grass to the top of the hill, from where we had a marvellous view of the whole Panama Canal. It was late evening, and the twinkling lights made the area look like a distant fairyland.

Deck tennis, a fast and skilful game, became a favourite pastime during our free time. I enjoyed it and became fairly competent. The exercise and fresh air were very beneficial.

On a gloriously hot, sunny day with clear blue skies we anchored out in the harbour at Acapulco. It was possible to water-ski in the bay, so a group of us went ashore in a lifeboat in search of the necessary equipment. We found a willing Mexican with a speedboat and skis. I had tried water-skiing once before but wasn't sure that I could still do it. I can still remember the tremendous exhilaration of getting up on the skis and swishing far out in the bay right round the *Canberra* before returning to the beach, exhausted but content with my achievement.

A documentary film called *Women at Sea* was made during this long voyage. All female personnel were filmed doing their various duties. I was photographed at the children's parties, in the playroom, at deck sports and when supervising the children's swimming lessons. Of course, my family and friends were most interested to see the film when it was shown in cinemas some months later.

While we were at Los Angeles, I had a chance to visit Disneyland with two of the officers who had friends living near the port. These friends collected us from the ship and took us to their home for coffee, and we met their families. Later, a large group of us spent about three hours at Disneyland. The following day in the playroom the children could talk of nothing else. For them all, it had been an experience of a lifetime, and I could quite understand why.

We had a wonderful send-off from Los Angeles. On a beautiful sunny evening, hundreds of speedboats and sailing yachts followed us out of the harbour. As we sailed majestically ahead, shouts of "bon voyage" came over loudspeakers to passengers onboard from well-wishers onshore. A band played rousing music, and brightly coloured streamers were thrown. As we reached the outer harbour, all the boats following us started to hoot, as if to say good-bye. We replied with four long hoots, and at that moment the sun sank below the horizon.

At San Francisco Bay we passed under two of the largest bridges in the world:

The Golden Gate and the Oakland Bridges. San Francisco is built on a hill, and the famous cable cars run straight up and down the hill's wide streets. The surrounding country is mountainous and very beautiful. The skyline, with high skyscrapers, is fascinating. The first view of the city from the harbour was breathtaking.

As usual, in American ports we were welcomed with a flotilla of little boats; since the *Canberra* was one of the largest liners to berth there, it always caused a great deal of excitement. Although the majority of passengers were going to New Zealand or Australia on this long voyage, some embarked or disembarked at each port we visited. Thus, new faces would appear amongst the children in the playroom.

I celebrated my twenty-ninth birthday on the day we arrived in Vancouver. The autumn colours were at their best, the maples and beeches glorious in the crisp, cold sunshine. Mountain ranges surrounded the large harbour. The radio officers told me that I should expect a cable call at midday. My mother's voice was extremely clear, and it was marvellous to have a chat.

The officers presented me with a large card that read, "Happy Birthday to the Hostess with the Mostest". There was a sketch with the signatures of all my friends onboard, as well as a pile of cards and letters from family and friends at home waiting for me when we berthed. Although I was so far away, they had not forgotten me—thank goodness.

In the evening I gave a party and invited thirty guests. The festivities really got going at about ten o'clock when everyone had finished work. I decorated my cabin, the empty one next to it and our corridor with posters I had collected from the tourist office in Vancouver, and I used the totem poles, headdresses and the shrunken heads we had made for the last children's party. One of the barmen made me an excellent punch with a champagne base, which seemed to do down very well. Everyone turned up in civilian clothes, a nice change from the usual ship's uniform. We had a record player and a large selection of Beatles and other records. There was dancing and general merriment until about two in the morning. I went to bed content that I had spent one of my best birthdays ever.

We had nearly a week at sea between Vancouver and Honolulu, so we had another children's party. This time they all dressed as Indians. The weather at sea was not so good, so nearly all the children spent their days in the playroom.

I had to pinch myself to believe we really had arrived at Honolulu. The new first-class children's hostess, Maggie, and I were to divide the day off, so as soon as we berthed I set off for Waikiki Beach. I sunbathed in a quiet spot on the beach. It was a perfect day, sunny but not too hot. I watched, fascinated by the handsome, young, surfboarders hurtling to the beach on the crests of waves at amazing speeds; some surfers executed complicated turns and twists. I can still remember the brilliantly coloured surfboards and the deep tan of their athletic bodies.

After I had been there for some time, enjoying the sun and the lively beach, one of these tall blond surfers came striding towards me, in actual fact, to pick up his towel and clothes, which were a yard or two away from me. He gave me a friendly smile as he passed and said, "Hi, what a great day." "Yes, isn't it marvellous?" I replied, sounding very English. "Well," he said, "it sounds as if you are a long way from home." Then he laid his towel out near mine and flopped down on the sandy beach. I explained that I was working on the *Canberra* and that we had berthed that morning.

It was the start of a very easy friendship. His name was Don, and he was a student at the Hawaiian university. He then offered me a lift on his motorbike back to the ship. This seemed a good idea, so I accepted.

I returned to Honolulu four more times. Each time Don met me at the gangway with a lei (a garland of flowers), as is the custom in Hawaii. On the back of his motorbike he took me to many interesting places and unspoilt beaches around the island. We had some delicious meals together in the evenings before he returned me safely to the ship. At one particular barbecue restaurant on the beach we cooked our own large tender steaks on charcoal grills and then helped ourselves to an enormous selection of salads and sauces. We sat at a little table drinking red wine under a straw umbrella on the moonlit beach with the sound of the waves on the sand. At the time I could not think of anything more perfect. But Don was just a good friend, and we were not in love. That was to come much later in my life.

The *Canberra* then had another long stretch at sea before reaching Auckland. I was sorry to say good-bye to the disembarking families. Children bound for Australia embarked, and as it was a very busy changeover day, I did not go ashore.

It was great to return to Sydney, for by now I knew the harbour well. A migrant family I had met on my first voyage met me on the quay. The children looked so well and happy and seemed to have grown inches. I spent the day at their home. The father, a qualified doctor, was now a general practitioner in Sydney. His wife had made new friends, and the children loved their schools. This move was thus a great success for each of them.

Next on the *Canberra's* itinerary was a cruise from Sydney to Auckland, Honolulu, Vancouver, San Francisco and Los Angeles, then back to Auckland and Sydney. Many of the passengers were on a holiday cruise. The weather was good, and I had few children to look after. Many invitations came my way to go ashore at the various ports. This was a very carefree, happy period of my life, one which I shall never forget. We had three days in Sydney; two of which I was entertained by previous passengers; on the third, a group of us spent some time shopping and sightseeing.

After a round cruise—from Sydney to Auckland, Honolulu, the ports of the American east coast and then back to Sydney—we were prepared for our homeward journey via Melbourne, Fremantle, Colombo, Port Said, Piraeus, Naples and Gibraltar. We reached Southampton just after Christmas. I was very ready for a two-week break at home, after which I was off again for my last long voyage, this time to the Far East.

Chapter 9

MY LAST *CANBERRA* VOYAGE

After leave at home I decided to do one more voyage with the P & O Company, mainly because doing so would enable me to see Hong Kong and Japan. The *Canberra* was due to sail via the Suez Canal to Ceylon around the coast of Australia to Sydney, and then to New Zealand. From here she was to do a cruise calling at Nuku'alofa, Honolulu, Vancouver, San Francisco, Los Angeles, Honolulu, Yokohama, Kobe, Nagasaki, Hong Kong, then back to Sydney and Auckland, returning to Southampton via the Panama Canal. It all sounded too good to be true; there would be very few children in the tourist class, and I would be paid during a voyage round the world.

But I was now beginning to see that life at sea was pretty superficial and in some ways like one long holiday. I realised that two years of this carefree life would be enough. Many of the officers onboard were married with families. At the end of each trip there was constant change amongst ship's officers; good friends left and new faces appeared. Children in the playroom were always changing, too, as families embarked and disembarked. I was beginning to long for some stability.

Previous visits to the Suez Canal had been too hectic to spend much time ashore, but this time I was able to have the whole day off. As we berthed at Port Said, hundred of little bumboats surrounded the ship, offering souvenirs, portable radios, binoculars, and other small electrical or battery-run goods. The noise was incredible as these men shouted up to the passengers on the open decks to catch a rope. They would call out, "What do you want to buy, Mrs Macdonald?"—all the women were "Mrs Macdonald". I bought a good pair of Zenith binoculars for five pounds, a small portable radio and two rocking camel stools for my two goddaughters, Annabelle and Antonia. As baskets were pulled up and down the side of the ship, bargains were struck, goods delivered and the agreed amount of money sent back into lowered basket.

When we were eventually able to go ashore, I joined a group of passengers going to Cairo to see Tutankhamen's treasures at the museum and the pyramids. It was very hot and smelly when we finally emerged from our air-conditioned coach at the foot of the pyramids. We were directed to a queue of tourists awaiting camel rides. The camels were an ugly sight, dirty and unkempt. They flicked their tails continually to distract the flies. I am almost ashamed to admit that I did have a ride. The camel went down on its front knees, and I clambered on to the saddle between the humps. As the camel rose, I was thrown backwards and then forwards, but once it started to walk I was able to relax and look around. A young Egyptian held a rope attached to the camel's bridle and led us in a circle around the nearest pyramid. The actual climb up the steps of a pyramid to look inside was not pleasant, and crowds of beggars tried to touch us as we passed. I think we were all glad to return safely to the *Canberra*.

As the *Canberra* was to call at Aden, I had written to my school friend Penny. Her husband, Bob, was now stationed there, and Penny and the children were with him. Neither Penny nor I realised how difficult it would be to find each other amongst the crowds of Arabs and tourists. I spent a frustrating afternoon waiting on the landing stage. Feeling very disappointed, I decided at last to return to the ship. Halfway across the boat I was in passed a lifeboat going in the opposite direction. I suddenly heard someone shout my name. Looking over to the other boat, I was amazed to see Penny waving frantically. I signalled that I would return to the shore. At last we met! We settled in a little café, drinking strong Turkish coffee, oblivious to the world around us for the next hour. We caught up with each other's news, and I was relieved to be able to hand over the camel stool for Antonia, which I had carried under my arm for most of the day.

The next excitement on this voyage was when we sailed into Sydney Harbour and found that the British fleet was in. I had once seen the fleet in Portsmouth: warships of all kinds; destroyers, aircraft carriers and gunboats. We decided to hold an open-house officers' party the next evening in the officers' wardroom on the *Canberra*. We sent out invitations over the radio and to all the naval ships. They were quickly acknowledged and accepted.

We had no idea how many would turn up. At the appointed time about twenty dashing young officers arrived in immaculate naval uniform. We had a great party. I think they enjoyed it all as much as we did. During the evening we discovered that the mayor of Sydney and his council were to be at a reception onboard the naval flagship the following day. To our delight and surprise, two of the officers invited my friend Marianne and me to the reception.

An official car was sent to fetch us the next day. We had been given special passes to the naval docks. A rating had obviously been detailed to look out for us. He opened the car door and then escorted Marianne and me to the foot of the gangway. I started up the gangway first. About halfway up I heard a soft swearword and I looked back to find Marianne struggling. She had somehow managed to get the heel of her shoe jammed in one of the steps. As she gave one last frantic tug, her shoe fell off and landed on the quay below. Fortunately, an officer quickly recovered the shoe and returned it to Marianne. Once more we started on our upwards journey and at last reached the top, where we were greeted by the admiral.

It was most interesting being introduced to the Mayor of Sydney at the end of the party. We were invited to a supper and then to a nightclub. Our handsome escorts took us back to the *Canberra* in the early hours of the morning. We all had a marvellous time. Unfortunately, we sailed later that day. After we had been at sea almost two months we reached Japan. Yokohama was our first port of call. As we berthed, I could see mountains in the distance and the snow-covered peak of Mount Fuji.

The *Canberra's* assistant surgeon had asked me to go ashore on my day off duty. This was as well, for as soon as I was ashore I realised it would be very difficult to find my way about, as I could neither read nor speak Japanese. We found the railway station and took a train to Tokyo. There we found our way with the aid of a map.

I was intrigued by the shop signs, which ran up and down like banners rather than across the tops like our western ones. I wished I could understand the artistic and colourful Japanese writing. Smartly dressed people walked at great speed along the pavements, but very few women were out that morning. I had heard that china and silk were the things to buy. We found some excellent shops, and I bought a most attractive Noritake coffee set and a length of emerald green silk for my sister. I was very pleased with my purchase. In the evening six of us went ashore for a meal, and we were waited on by very pretty geisha girls.

Our next stop on the Japanese coast was at Kobe. We arrived at about seven in the morning. At 9.00, four of us were able to go ashore and join a tour going to Kyoto, the ancient capital of Japan. The coach took some time to get out of the modern, industrialised city and into the country. We passed a great many paddy fields with peasants at work and caught a glimpse of the new express train, which travels at about one hundred forty miles per hour. Kyoto itself is full of ancient buildings and many Buddhist shrines and temples. We were shown an old castle which had a beautiful Japanese garden with pagodas and flowering shrubs. Unfortunately, it was too late in the season for cherry blossoms. While we were at the castle, a crowd of school children arrived, all wearing the same smart uniform. We were told they were on a school outing. We lunched in a large hotel in the centre of Kyoto but were disappointed not to have local Japanese food—we were given roast beef, sprouts and roast potatoes! To make up for this, four of us from the ship went out for a meal in the evening. In a long barn-shaped room we sat on large cushions on the floor beside low tables and ate with chopsticks. High-pitched Japanese music and dancing was our entertainment. Our sukiyaki, strips of beef in a rather sweet soy sauce with all kinds of roots and vegetables, was cooked at the table. To this was added a raw egg—it was delicious.

One last stop in Japan was Nagasaki. I joined a tour going to the museum where the horrific effects of the atom bomb were on display. I felt I ought go and see the evidence of this terrible disaster. It was far worse than I could ever have imagined. I prayed, then and there, that this should never happen again.

On the trip from Japan to Hong Kong I had two adorable little Chinese girls in my playroom. They were very polite and spoke good English. One was three and the other five years old.

Visiting Hong Kong was the most exciting part of the voyage for me. I was lucky enough to have an old family friend working there; he had promised to look after me and show me round during our stay. My first memory of Keith was of waving good-bye to him as he drove off on his motorbike. During the war, I was about seven years old, both our families used to meet in a small village on the edge of Dartmoor. Keith had just been called up and was going off in his army uniform.

My next memory of Keith was when I was about fourteen; he arrived in a flashy little sports car at our thatched house in Andover and took me for a ride. We roared along at great speed with the roof down and the wind in our hair. As soon as I knew *Canberra* was going to call at Hong Kong, I wrote to him. I received a letter saying he would love to see me. I was to phone his number, and he would come and meet me at the Hilton Hotel.

We approached Hong Kong up a creek surrounded by high mountains and hills;

as we rounded the last bend, the modern skyscrapers tightly packed on the hillsides came into view. Here and there we could see squatters' houses, where the very poor lived. The *Canberra* had an amazing reception. Hundreds of junks came out to greet us, and some had musicians onboard. Gaily decorated with flags, these little boats, mostly laden with families, crowded round the ship. The father had a fishing net, and the mother manoeuvred the boat with a long pole. There were usually two or three small children, and occasionally the mother had a baby tied in a sling on her back. We threw down plastic dolls and small toys to some of these children.

I was off duty for three of the four days we spent at Hong Kong. As planned, I made my way to the Hilton Hotel and rang Keith. Soon he was striding in through the hotel doors. He was tall, slim, tanned and wearing glasses. I recognised his smiling face instantly. We made our way to the ferry and crossed to the island. We found Keith's MG and drove up the peak to where some friends of his lived. Mervyn and Kathleen's flat was near the top and had a wonderful view over the harbour. After a drink the four of us set off round the island to a fishing village called Aberdeen. There, hundreds of people lived in little boats on the water's edge. Because of the shortage of any kind of living accommodation, families slept onboard—in shifts. But the amazing thing was they did not look hungry or unhappy. Wherever we walked, little boys begged us for coins, and they had such enchanting smiles and happy faces that one could not fend them off.

After parking the car, we walked along a landing stage to a little boat with wicker chairs, and two women propelled us with long poles to a floating restaurant. We arrived in time to see the end of a wedding reception, where a very loud band was playing amazing music. Fortunately, the noise soon stopped. The bride looked very lovely in a very ornate wedding gown. I was told that by custom she was not allowed to speak to anyone during the ceremony.

Once on the floating restaurant we were escorted to a room with large fish tanks round the walls. The fish on the menu were still happily swimming about. Mervyn knew what to order. He chose enormous king-size prawns, which were then caught in front of our eyes. Then a large, long fish was caught. Finally, a very large crab was pulled out and hustled away to its death. As we sat waiting in the ornate Chinese dining room of our meal to be cooked, we saw firecrackers being set off from one of the nearby boats. Also, while we waited for our dinner, I tried one of a large assortment of little dishes with sauces and peppers on a piece of bread. I nearly set my mouth on fire! It served me right for being so greedy and impatient! I really thought my mouth would never be normal again!

Before we began dinner a hot-scented flannel was given to each of us. First we had shark's fin soup, which was really delicious, followed by the king prawns, which we peeled and ate with our fingers. We each had differently coloured and decorated chopsticks for the side dishes of rice. There was China tea or shandy to drink. Just as we were preparing to leave the restaurant, there was a heavy storm with lightning and thunder. It had been a very hot and humid evening, and by the time we got back to the car my hair was hanging limp and straight. Keith took me back on the ferry, and I was glad to return to my air-conditioned cabin on the *Canberra* for a refreshing shower.

The next day Keith had to work, and I was on duty in the playrooms; but in the evening I was able to entertain Keith to dinner onboard in the first-class dining room. Later I took him on a tour of the ship. Our last day in Hong Kong happened to be a Saturday, so Keith was not working. He arrived at the *Canberra* with a streaming cold. Nonetheless, he was determined to take me by train to the new territories and on to the Chinese border. We had a wonderful day together, and the trip gave me a good glimpse of the countryside. As we approached the border we passed field after field, where peasants were tending the rice crops. They were all wearing the traditional uniform—blue working clothes and wide-brimmed coolie hats. I noticed the peasants were all women, expect for the occasional man who seemed to be in charge of a gang of workers. We returned to Hong Kong, where we spent the afternoon shopping. In the evening Keith took me out for another excellent dinner, and then it was time to say good-bye, as the *Canberra* was to sail very early next morning. It had been a marvellous four days.

I was once again busy with nearly two hundred children to amuse. One morning a very worried stewardess came to me. A three-year-old boy called Billy Brown was rolling round the playroom floor with what appeared to be agonising stomach pain. I went immediately to see him and found a very pale, sweaty little boy screaming and drawing up his legs as he rocked from side to side.

I knew Billy quite well. He was a lively, likeable child with an older brother and sister who were not in the playroom at the time. His parents had originally emigrated from England to Sydney, but after two or three years they had decided to move on to Canada.

Something was seriously wrong with Billy, so I picked him up and took him straight to the ship's hospital. There the ship's surgeon examined him. I was able to leave him in the capable hands of my friend, the nursing sister, and went to find his parents. By the time we returned Billy was much calmer, having been given painkillers and a sedative.

At this time, the *Canberra* was sailing from Auckland to Honolulu, we still had twenty-four hours to go before reaching the Hawaiian Islands. The ship's surgeon was worried about Billy's condition, and after a conference with the captain it was decided to arrange by ship's radio for an ambulance to be waiting to take Billy straight ashore to the modern hospital for special paediatric investigations. As I was a children's trained nurse, I was asked to escort him.

Billy was cared for in the ship's hospital until we berthed at Honolulu. Because of immigration rules, unfortunately his parents were unable to go ashore with him. We dressed him in his pyjamas, dressing gown and slippers, packed a bag with a few necessities and tried to explain to him what was going to happen.

The ambulance's emergency team came onboard very quickly, and Billy was taken off the ship on a stretcher. He was a very brave little boy and clung to my hand; at times this was difficult, especially down the narrow gangway. Once he was settled in the ambulance we shot off at a tremendous speed with the sirens screaming. He had a police escort, and we soon reached the hospital. After a short wait in casualty he was seen by a paediatric surgeon. Billy had a thorough examination followed by blood tests and x-rays. All this brought back memories of Great Ormond Street to me.

Eventually the paediatric surgeon came to talk to me, he told me Billy was to be admitted to the children's ward and would have emergency abdominal surgery later that day. He handed me a letter which would authorise Billy's parents to come to the hospital immediately in order to sign the operation consent form. They would then be able to stay with Billy until after the operation.

The police took me back to the *Canberra* and waited while I informed the parents, who were then taken to see Billy. Meanwhile, I looked after the two older children onboard the ship. This ordeal was most distressing, especially as we were due to sail again the next evening.

While I had been at the hospital, my friend Don (the university student) had, as usual, come to meet me when we berthed at Honolulu. My friends had told him where I was, and he returned in the evening to take me ashore for dinner. He was as concerned as I was when I told him about Billy, so we decided to go and visit him in the hospital the following morning.

The operation was for a blockage, and a section of Billy's intestine was removed. When Don and I visited the hospital the next morning, Billy was in intensive care and was only allowed to see his parents. Although his mother and father were much relieved when the surgeon told them the operation had been a success, they were most distressed at the thought of having to leave Billy in the hospital on his own while the rest of the family went on to Canada, but they had no choice. Don promised he would do everything he could to help Billy. Don kept his word and went to the Honolulu newspaper office to tell them about Billy and his family. An appeal was set up to help when he recovered. Don also organised a rota of his university friends to go and visit Billy in the hospital.

When I returned to Southampton nearly a month later there was a letter from Don telling me that Billy had made a remarkable recovery. The people of Honolulu had raised sufficient money in the "Billy Brown" appeal to fly him to join his family in Vancouver.

Chapter 10

BACK TO PAEDIATRIC NURSING

Clearing my cabin and leaving the *Canberra* was a mammoth operation. During my two years at sea, I had acquired and purchased a great many things, especially during the last voyage around the world. Each item reminded me of different adventures or places I had visited. The colourful onion-shaped basket from the straw market now serves as a laundry basket. The round wicker table with black wrought-iron legs, which I gave to my mother has been used in the garden ever since. The camel carpet from Cairo was commandeered by my son. There was also my picture of the sunset at Honolulu, which had been specially painted for me by Don.

My mother was flabbergasted when she saw the packing cases and piles of luggage which somehow had to be taken home. We stacked it all in the car, and I left the *Canberra* for the last time with feelings of sadness.

Readjusting to life on land took quite a while. For many years, I would occasionally dream that I was back onboard the *Canberra*. I would feel the movement of the ship and hear the waves swishing against her great white hull; sometimes I recalled the feeling of near panic at the start of a big children's party.

I spent the first few weeks catching up with all of my old friends. I bought a yellow Mini and dashed around. Each week I scanned the *Nursing Times* and the *Nursing Mirror* for vacant appointments. My paediatric nursing skills and expertise would, I knew, be very rusty by now. Eventually, I saw an advertisement for a job which sounded like just what I needed.

The Brompton Chest Hospital, London, was starting nine-month, postgraduate paediatric intensive-care courses. All applicants had to have a Registered Sick Children's Nurse qualification and have at least one year of experience as a staff nurse. I applied immediately and was asked to go for an interview the following week.

Jo Sterry was now working at The Florence Nightingale Foundation in London. She shared a flat in Earl's Court with a friend named Rosemary Esch. It was years since Jo and I had seen much of each other, but, as with all really close friends, it only seemed like yesterday that we had celebrated her twenty-first birthday at the Wimbledon Tennis Club. I telephoned her, and an amazed, giggly Jo answered, "Yes, of course! You must come and stay with us for the interview. What fun! We'll have a really good natter."

I drove to London on the day before the interview, found Jo's flat and settled in. We had a wonderful evening catching up with each other's news. Like myself, Jo had not married. After spending time as a nanny and cook in the States, she had returned as an administrator to the nursing world in England at the Nursing

Charitable Foundation, which sponsored postgraduate nurses in specialised fields for scholarships.

My interview went well. The hospital on Brompton Road is a very old establishment specialising in the care of chest diseases. They hoped to have about ten students on the course. The idea was twofold: to train more staff in paediatric intensive care and to enable the hospital to staff the children's ward with competent nurses. The first course was to commence the following month. The students would work shifts on the ward for five days and have half a day of lectures given by consultants and senior nursing staff; students would have off the remaining day and a half. I came away hoping that I had secured a place on the course. I liked everything I had seen, and it was just what I needed to get back into paediatric care.

Back at Jo's flat, I met Rosemary for the first time. "Where will you live?" she asked.

This was quite a problem, as I had been told at the Brompton Chest Hospital that there was no nursing accommodation available. Rosemary suggested that her mother might let me have a room. After a phone call to Rosemary's mother, it was arranged for me to go to see her the following day.

Mrs Esch lived in a Victorian-terraced house with a walled garden at the back. She lived on her own and said that she would be delighted to have a friend of Jo and Rosemary's to stay. The room, small but adequate, was not really set up as a bed-sitter, but I knew that I would have all main meals at the hospital. It was just what I required, and the rent was low.

Everything now depended on whether I would be accepted. I was jubilant when, about a week later, I received a letter confirming that I had secured a place on the course. I was due to start in a fortnight.

I loved living in West Kensington. When I was at the Great Ormond Street and The Middlesex Hospitals, I lived in the centre of the city. West Kensington was more like a village, and it had its own church, post office, shops and pubs. I began to recognise the faces I saw daily when going to and coming from the tube stations. Weekends in West Kensington were particularly pleasant.

I remember very little about the actual course. As a group, we did not make friends, as we were always on different shifts and hardly ever ran into one another. The paediatric ward was small. It was at the top of the old hospital building and consisted of eight large cubicle rooms, four on either side of the main corridor, the sister's office and the usual utility rooms.

Most of the patients were newborn babies with congenital heart disease who came from all over England. There was an incubator in each cubicle and all the necessary equipment for emergency admissions. After cardiac catherisation to diagnose the defect, x-rays and other essential tests, most of these babies were taken to the operating theatre for lifesaving surgery. Sometimes they were there for hours; one never knew whether the surgeons would be successful or not. It was then our job to nurse these tiny babies, who were never left alone. Each day the students relieved one another throughout the twenty-four hours until the babies were out of danger. The senior registrar was very tall, rather untidy and not much older than myself; he had been born and bred in Ireland. For the first few weeks I was really afraid of him. He would stride the ward with his white coat flapping and fire curt questions at us about the little babies in our care. He certainly did not suffer fools gladly. I noticed he was nearly always on call in the hospital. But as I got to know him better and understand his brusque manner, I grew to admire and, indeed, to like him.

A dedicated and very ambitious young doctor, the senior registrar could not bear for things to go wrong and to lose a baby. He had enormous hands but sensitive and deft fingers. I often watched him beside an incubator, with an arm through each side window. He was so tall he had to bend over all the time. In a white mask and gown he would spend an hour or more trying to get a minute catheter into a small vein of a tiny, seven-pound newborn baby. He had incredible patience and expertise.

One morning my alarm clock failed to go off, and I overslept. I woke with a start to discover that it was nearly time for the beginning of the morning shift at the hospital. I had no time for breakfast or even a drink. After hastily dressing, I ran to the tube station; luckily, a train arrived almost immediately and whisked me to Brompton Road. I dashed to the hospital and up the two flights of stairs to the children's ward. The ward sister greeted me with, "You are half an hour late, Miss Gedge, but you are just in time to go and help the doctor with a very tricky procedure."'

I took a deep breath and tried to control my heaving chest as I went into the cubicle where the senior registrar was already waiting for me. In a trance, I washed my hands, put on a gown and mask and took up my position on the opposite side of the incubator. My job was to hold the tiny baby's leg completely still whilst the doctor set up a lifesaving intravenous infusion. I knew it could take a very long time, and I would be unable to move once the procedure got under way. I prayed inwardly that I would be able to cope. I was foolish. I should have told the sister or the doctor that I had had nothing to eat or drink that morning, but at the time I was too scared.

The baby was very ill indeed. His colour was poor, and he had a very weak pulse, which meant it would be extremely difficult to find a vein big enough to insert the catheter. After about three-quarters of an hour of fruitless attempts, I began to feel very cold, and sweat started pouring down my forehead. Desperately, I tried to switch my weight from one leg to another, but my attempt was no good. I knew I was going to faint. Vaguely, I heard myself say, "Sorry, but I've got to go." I remember staggering out of the cubicle and calling the sister in a pathetically feeble voice. After that I fainted. When I came round, the sister and the rest of the nursing staff were most sympathetic, but I wondered what the doctor would say to me. To my surprise, later that morning he came to reassure me that the baby was looking much better. He asked how I was and gave me a comforting smile.

I came to enjoy working with the senior registrar, and he taught me much. Gradually, I discovered that he had a great sense of humour, and towards the end of the course I even went out with him once or twice. There were occasions when he would tease me unmercifully. I'd love to know what happened to him. My guess is that somewhere he has reached the top of the medical profession.

We students were awarded a diploma at the end of the nine-month course. I now felt ready to apply for a paediatric sister or senior staff nurse's post. I stayed on in my West Kensington bed-sitter whilst keeping an eye on the weekly nursing magazine.

As it as the start of the summer, London was full of tourists. I had the bright idea of running my own business, which I decided to call Children's Tours of London. I had some cards printed and displayed them in several of the large West End hotels. Mrs Esch allowed me to put her telephone number on the cards. I had a fair number of enquiries and did, in fact, escort children to places like the Tower of London, Madame Tussaud's, the planetarium and the science museum. I charged a ridiculously small sum for this service and responsibility. In those days, rules of child care and insurance were very lax; it amazes me now to think that parents, who knew virtually nothing about me, allowed their young children to go off in my care on trips round London.

Fortunately, by the end of the summer I found the advertisement I had been looking for, a relief sister's post on the paediatric wards at the Radcliffe Infirmary, Oxford. I applied, was interviewed and got the job. But once again I had the problem of finding accommodation.

I knew that Liz from the *Canberra* now had a teaching post in a primary school near the Cowley Motor works, Oxford. I also knew that she lived in a bed-sitter in a large house on Woodstock Road, also in Oxford. But she was about to move nearer home before getting married and would be leaving her bed-sitter just about the time that I was due to start work at the Radcliffe Infirmary. It turned out to be an amazingly convenient coincidence, and I was able to take over her room.

From the moment I started working on the children's wards, I realised how privileged I was to join such a dedicated, hardworking and caring paediatric team. The post of relief sister was a new one, and it entailed working between the medical and surgical children's wards, which were situated one above the other in the main building.

Dr Hugh Ellis was in charge of the paediatric department. He was a kindly, plump, comfortable person. No problem or difficulty was too much trouble for him; he had endless patience. His speciality was children with leukaemia. Even though he was a senior consultant, he would come in to see a sick child at any time of the day or night.

The children and their parents had complete confidence in him, and they loved him. Every Christmas, Dr Ellis and his delightful wife invited the entire paediatric team to their beautifully decorated home for a traditional dinner at the end of a busy Christmas Day.

Dr Brian Bower was a medical paediatric consultant specialising in neurology. He was younger than Dr Ellis and was a tall, handsome man, quietly spoken, with slightly greying hair. He, too, had great patience and would spend endless time examining and testing a child who had some obscure neurological problem. These two consultants shared the twenty-four medical beds on the ward, taking turns to be on call.

Downstairs, Mr Malcolm Gough was the senior surgical paediatric consultant. He was in his early forties and was a brilliant and ambitious surgeon. He carried out a wide range of children's operations but specialised in neonatal surgery, correcting many different congenital defects.

Then there were the senior registrars. Dr Douglas Pickering specialised in cardiology and was an expert at diagnosis using cardiac cathersation. I soon discovered that he had met his wife, Flora, while he was working as a doctor on the same P & O ship where she was the children's hostess. Downstairs, Dr David Hide was the senior surgical registrar he specialised in children with hydrocephalus and eventually formed a special unit attached to the surgical ward to care for these children.

Drs Gough, Pickering and Hide had young families and it wasn't long before I was being asked to baby-sit while their parents went out. I loved these evenings with healthy, normal children, and my experience as a children's hostess came in useful, as the younger ones always wanted to make something before going to bed. Baby-sitting also gave me a chance to get to know the doctors and their families away from the hospital.

I was lucky to work with, and relieve, two experienced and friendly sisters. Judith Bywater, who had trained at St Thomas' Hospital, London, was in charge of Leopold Medical. She looked very attractive in her blue sister's uniform, with its white starched apron, and her short, dark, wavy hair tucked under her pleated cap. The children loved her, and she ran a happy, efficient ward, training the student nurses in paediatrics as they worked with her. Annie Ballegooigen was sister on Leopold Surgical Ward. She was a lively, amusing character and an excellent sister who was very popular with the doctors, nurses and children in her care. I relieved these two sisters on their days off. I learnt to take responsibility for a ward in my temporary care and to make decisions. It was excellent training, especially as all the members of the experienced paediatric team were willing to spend time teaching me.

Being on the general medical and surgical children's wards was a new experience for me. All my sick children's nursing at Great Ormond Street Hospital had been very specialised. I had not nursed everyday illnesses like asthmatic cases or children with very high temperatures caused by viral infection, meningitis or urinary infections. I remember one little boy being rushed in with croup; he was in a very bad way, because his trachea had swollen so much that air was no longer able to pass through it. The emergency team was called, and he was immediately intubated and given oxygen. When his condition had improved sufficiently, he was taken to theatre to have a small tube inserted through his neck into the trachea (a tracheostomy) to insure that he would have a good airway. About ten days later when the infection had responded to antibiotics and the child was no longer ill, the tube was removed, and he breathed normally again. He was a little mischief and a real character when he was up and about again. It was difficult to believe we had nearly lost him.

Neither had I nursed children who had routine appendicectomy or hernia operations or who were in traction or plaster after accidents. I soon realised that many of the children who had been in accidents could be very naughty, because they were bored and did not feel ill. Fortunately, there were teachers and play leaders to teach and amuse them in the mornings, and there was visiting everyday.

I served as the relief sister for two years. During the second year, I followed with great interest plans to make a Special-Care unit which would be attached to the existing surgical ward. The consultants made me feel that I might be considered as a sister for this new unit. I became increasingly excited. This was exactly the sort of paediatric nursing in which I wanted to specialise.

Chapter 11

A MONTH IN AMERICA AND CANADA
OBSERVING PAEDIATRIC UNITS

In 1969, towards the end of my two years as relief sister on the paediatric wards at the Radcliffe Infirmary, I was introduced to Mr Alf Gunning, the cardiac consultant surgeon. He was a short, stocky and extremely fit man, with a slight South-African accent. I had heard he was very talented and had carried out lengthy heart surgery on adults. In conversation I found out that he was keen to have the chance to operate on children with congenital heart defects. At that time children in the cardiac department were sent to Birmingham or London for surgery because of a lack of intensive-care facilities at the Radcliffe Infirmary. He was as interested in the progress of the Special-Care unit as I was. He discovered that I had originally trained at Great Ormond Street Hospital, where he had spent time working as a surgeon. He was also interested in my paediatric intensive-care nursing course at Brompton Chest Hospital. I found Mr. Gunning extremely easy to talk to and confessed that I was very much hoping to be considered as a possible sister for the new unit.

By now I had an idea at the back of my mind that I might resign my post as relief sister and go to America and Canada for a month at my own expense in order to visit as many paediatric intensive-care units as possible. I mentioned this plan to Mr Gunning who was most encouraging; the experience could only be of help to me.

So a few days later I decided to throw caution to the wind; I handed in my resignation. This meant I would finish being relief sister at the end of the month. After I had explained what I was proposing to do, my landlady very kindly said she would keep my room for me until I returned to England.

My first move was to write to the matrons of the Boston Children's Hospital, the Toronto Children's Hospital and the Foothills Hospital at Calgary. In my letters I explained my reasons for going and asked if it would be possible to observe some major cardiac surgery and, more importantly, spend time in their intensive-care units.

Another reason for going to Canada at this time was that Douglas Pickering, the senior registrar, had gone to Toronto to spend a year in the cardiac unit of the children's hospital. Both he and his wife, Flora, had given me an open invitation to stay with them if I ever came to Toronto.

The replies from all three matrons were most encouraging. Boston Children's Hospital said they could offer me everything I had requested and accommodate me in their nurses' home for three nights. The other two matrons agreed to my visiting and observing their intensive-care units. When I had finalised my plans, they asked me to inform them of the dates I would arrive.

By this time I was extremely excited. The only remaining problem was whether

I could afford the flight. Amazingly, I found an advertisement at the back of the *Nursing Mirror* for return economy flights to New York at the incredibly low cost of sixty nine pounds. I made enquiries, found the details were correct and booked a flight. Now I really felt I was halfway to America.

Friends who had visited the States several times told me about Greyhound buses. With a British passport, you could get a monthly ticket in England for forty-one pounds (approximately ninety-nine dollars). This ticket would be valid for any journey in Canada and America. So I made last-minute arrangements, chose clothes to take and packed. Everyone at the Radcliffe Infirmary was most supportive, and very soon I was on my way to New York.

My first impression of America was disastrous. I had to take a taxi from the Kennedy Airport to the coach station. In my naivety I forgot I was not in London, and on arrival at the coach station I got out of the taxi and handed the driver a large amount of dollar bills, as I had no small change. To my utter dismay the wretched man snatched the notes and drove off at high speed. The incident certainly taught me a lesson.

Somehow I found the correct Greyhound bus. It took me eighty miles north to where I had planned to stay with friends who used to live opposite my mother's house in Winchester. Tom, who worked at IBM in England for a time, had made me promise I would go and visit him and his family if I ever got to America. Now I accepted his kind invitation. Tom and his family lived way out in the country in a house, which was lovely, despite the awful stink which seemed to prevade the place. I was told it was the smell of skunks.

After staying three nights, I climbed aboard another Greyhound bus for the second stage of my journey to Boston. I loved that old university city, with its distinctive English flavour. Having found my way to the children's hospital, I was shown a room in the nurse's home, which I could have for three dollars a night.

I spent two whole fascinating days at the hospital and had a senior nurse to accompany me the whole time. We went to two most interesting lectures on paediatric cardiac surgery given by very eminent surgeons. In addition, I spent a lot of time observing the intensive-care units and even watched operations in progress.

The operations were performed in a special kind of chamber where the air was compressed, rather like it is in a submarine. This enabled the baby patient to have a very concentrated oxygen flow. The doctors and nurses had to be specially prepared before entering this chamber, and they had to be slowly decompressed after the operation so that they did not suffer from the bends. All infants undergoing heart surgery were operated on in this chamber, but the air was not always compressed.

During my second evening in Boston a Scottish and a Canadian nurse took me out to dinner at a fabulous restaurant which looked just like a ship. It was famous for seafood and was called Anthony's Pick 4. The entrance door was opened by a pirate with a wooden leg. Cocktails and coffee were served on the splendidly furnished and decorated ship, and meals were eaten in the attractive dining room on the adjacent pier. We had a wonderful evening. My nursing companions were such fun, and at the end of the evening they escorted me safely back to the nurses' home, where I spent my last night in Boston.

After thanking the matron for all her help and saying farewell to her staff, I set off for the coach station. This time the Greyhound bus was bound for Toronto. The journey took the whole day.

All the Pickering family came to meet me at the Toronto bus station. Douglas, Flora and their three delightful children, David, Caroline and Elizabeth Jane, who was two years old. It was good to see them all again. David and Caroline were attending school in Toronto and had already acquired slight Canadian accents. Elizabeth Jane was very bright and mischievous. Their attractive flat on the fifteenth floor of an apartment block had a very splendid view.

I stayed in Toronto for a week. The children's hospital was a wonderful place and in many ways reminded me of Great Ormond Street. Light, airy and cheerful, this hospital had been designed throughout specifically for children and their parents. I was amused to see that the hospital's playroom and play-lady routine was almost exactly like ours had been at the Radcliffe Infirmary.

I spent three days on the intensive-care unit, which was fabulously modern and space saving. I made countless notes and drawings of their layout. The staff let me have pamphlets with information on various pieces of equipment I had never seen before. I discovered that they had dilemmas and difficulties just like we had in England; and as far as I could see, they had not really solved their problems with infant respirators any more than we had.

The intensive-care unit was extremely busy and had a very large turnover of patients. I was able to see at least two major cases return from theatre each day, including the Mustard operation, for transposition of the great vessels and total correction of Fallot's tetralogy. All the doctors and nursing staff were very helpful and explained all the procedures of the nursing care as they were performing them. I was glad I had taken the course at Brompton Chest Hospital, for as a result I could understand most of what the doctors and nurses told me.

Towards the end of the first day in the unit I was privileged to meet Mr Mustard himself when he came to check his patients. He had invented the Mustard operation, which corrected the blood flow in a child where the aorta and vena cavae are transposed. With this condition, the oxygenated blood and the venous blood each go into the wrong side of the heart, so that the child has no satisfactory circulation of oxygenated blood, which results in a poor quality of life and prognosis. Mr Mustard enquired if I would like to go into the theatre and watch him perform an operation the following morning.

Observing the operation was an amazing experience. I stood almost next to Mr Mustard, and he explained each step of the operation as he progressed. The patient was a three-year-old boy with a poor prognosis. Later in the day I went to see the child in the intensive-care unit and was surprised to find him awake and with a good colour. He was attached to a great number of tubes and monitors, and his mother was sitting at his bedside holding his hand.

During one of my days at the hospital, I was taken to see the neonatal floor, which at that time was the largest unit in the world. There were over seventy babies, most of them in incubators, several weighing under three pounds; they were all nationalities.

During the week, I had one day off from observing hospitals and took a

Greyhound bus to Niagara Falls. It was a gloriously hot day, and the falls really did come up to my expectations. The thunder and roar of the falling water was terrific. I saw the falls from three points: from a tower at the top, from a road at the side and then—the most exciting view—during a tour in the caves below with the full force of the water in front of us. We had to wear heavy mackintoshes.

While I was in Toronto, I visited relatives of one of my school friends. They had a lovely house and garden on the outskirts of the town. I spent a very happy evening with this family and discovered that my host was a kidney specialist at Toronto General Hospital. His wife, Jane, joined me for lunch the next day, and we explored Yorkville, which was a fascinating area filled with little art galleries, boutiques and handicraft shops.

I was thoroughly spoilt all the time I was in Toronto. Douglas and Flora took me out on my last evening. First, we rode in an outside elevator up an incredibly high skyscraper to have cocktails at the top. I was glad I have a good head for heights. Then we had an excellent meal at a French restaurant amongst the bustling night life of that exciting modern city.

From Toronto I took a Greyhound bus right across southern Canada. In the next seat was a young lad called John, who was about twenty, tall, strong, good looking and English. He was looked for a job in Canada and hoping to emigrate if he liked the life. He had started at Montreal, but as he was unable to speak French, he had no luck there. He was great company and most amusing. Every time the bus stopped he would leap off the bus to make hurried enquiries about jobs. My journey across Canada was to take me through Ontario and the Prairie Provinces to Calgary at the foothills of the Rocky Mountains. It took two days and two nights of solid driving at approximately seventy-five miles per hour along the Trans-Canada Highway. Many, like myself, did the whole journey on one bus, sleeping as much as possible at night in order to avoid the cost of overnight accommodation. We stopped every three to four hours for refreshments and loo visits, also to change drivers and sometimes to change a few passengers. These stops gave us a chance to stretch our legs and get some fresh air.

Ontario was mostly forested, and we passed a great number of rivers and lakes. Lake Superior was enormous: we seemed to go along its shores for hours. At one stop in a town surrounded by forest John shot off in search of a job. I began to get really anxious for when the bus was nearly ready to depart, he had still not reappeared. At the last minute he came dashing up, and with a broad grin he shouted through the window to me. "Hey, I got a job! I'm going to be a logger!" I congratulated him and then almost immediately the bus started moving, and we were waving frantically to each other like old friends. We had only known each other for a few hours, but I found myself thinking and worrying about John for some time after we left him. A Canadian passenger explained to me what a logger was. It sounded like decidedly dangerous hard work. Loggers steer the long tree trunks down the fast-flowing rivers, and at times the loggers have actually to ride on the logs. But apparently the pay was quite good, and John would be trained as an apprentice by experienced loggers.

Next we crossed the Prairie Provinces, the flat wheat fields around Winnipeg. Then the terrain gradually changed to moorland. I saw many granaries and elevators, usually situated near the railway lines, as well as oil pumps, which worked continuously day and night. There were herds of cattle grazing. When we stopped at places like Medicine Hat, Swift Current or Moose Jaw, I saw cowboys just like those I had seen in films at home; some were on horseback. I also met Habinats, a group who immigrated to Canada from the Ukraine; they are now rich farmers living in colonies. The Habinat ladies wore long dresses and hid their hair under caps; the men dressed in black.

Eventually, we arrived at Calgary. I had no accommodation arranged but had heard of the "Friends of Canada Association", a network of people who are prepared to give tourists bed and breakfast at short notice and for little money. One of my fellow bus travellers had given me a leaflet about this association. There were several telephone numbers of "Friends" to ring in Calgary. The first person I called said she could put me up for the night. She was a widow living on her own in a three-bedroom bungalow and seemed pleased to have unexpected company for the night. The room she offered me was small but adequate and had a very comfortable bed, which I could hardly wait to get into after such a long journey on the bus.

There was a very modern hospital in Calgary, located in a superb position on a hill overlooking the town on the one side and the Rocky Mountains in the distance on the other. The matron was most helpful, and a senior nurse showed me round the up-to-date and attractive paediatric unit.

I stayed two days in Calgary and then continued on my journey. My plan was to have a few days off in Banff, an attractive ski resort in the mountains. I found a small guest house, where the owners were kind and friendly. The weather was perfect, with cloudless blue skies, and as it was nearly the end of the season, the resort was not crowded. One ski area called Sunshine was still open. From a small cafe at the foot of the run I watched enviously as skiers swished past me.

Another day I took a trip up to Lake Louise. I had been determined to do this, as one of the mountains is named Mount Lefroy after one of my mothers' relations. Unfortunately, Lake Louise was still frozen and looked more like a snow field, but I found Mount Lefroy to be an impressive sight at the corner of the lake.

One evening my hosts suggested taking me up the narrow track behind the guest house to the local tip to look for wild animals. It was dusk when we set off up the hill in their land rover. Gary, their six-year-old son, came with us. It was bitterly cold that evening, so he wore a thick tweed coat and a hat with ear flaps to keep him warm. Near the top of the hill we arrived at a large circular area surrounded by thick bushes and trees. At one end was the local tip, which was an enormous rubbish dump. We sat very still in the land rover and peered ahead as darkness fell. It was several minutes before anything happened, then I felt Gary's hand touch my arm, and he pointed silently towards some bushes to the right of us. Two wolverine were nervously sniffing at the ground. Then, as if feeling more confident, they approached the dump and started to scrounge for food. Before long they were joined by some coyotes. They all seemed quite unaware of our presence.

We returned to the guest house, where I was asked to join the rest of the family for their evening meal. By the time we had finished Gary was yawning his head off. On the way home in the land rover he had made me promise to read him a story before he went to sleep. Which tale should he choose? Of course it had to be

"Little Red Riding Hood" with the big bad wolf. By the time I had finished the tale, little Gary was fast asleep. After a really good rest from Greyhound buses and a brief holiday in Banff, I turned my head towards home, catching yet another bus which was to take me east across the northern states of America. I spent a night in Winnipeg, staying at the YWCA, which was comfortable, convenient and quite close to the coach station. I had to change buses in Chicago. The coach station there was very scary and the only place on my entire trip where I felt alone and frightened. I had to wait nearly two hours for my connection, and there were a number of very suspicious characters in the waiting rooms. Armed police patrolled the bus station continuously, and at least three times they accused me of loitering. I had to explain that I was waiting for a Greyhound bus connection. I was extremely relieved when we finally drove out of the city.

When I did talk to Americans in the cafes or on the bus, I realised there was tremendous tension about the Vietnam War and Cambodia, and they all feared anything could flare up at any moment. Our route took us through Detroit, London (in Canada), Buffalo and eventually back to Toronto. Returning to Douglas and Flora's flat was like going home. The whole family gave me a great welcome. Douglas introduced me to his boss, Professor Keith, and showed me round the cardiology department.

By this time I had only a few days left on my monthly Greyhound bus ticket, so I decided to head back to New York. Now spring, the countryside was beautiful with flowering trees and spring flowers. A friend from Great Ormond Street had given me a contact in New York. I had telephoned her from Toronto, and she had offered to meet my bus. As I got off the bus, she greeted me, "Hallo. You must be Mary from England." As it was evening and I was starving, we went straight to an excellent restaurant renowned for its seafood. Once again, I was amazed at how well we got on.

I stayed the night in New York YWCA, which was clean, comfortable and centrally located. Then I had one day to explore New York. I took a three-hour trip round Manhattan on a boat. In the afternoon I went on a tram and tried desperately to follow my map of the city so that I would know when to get off. I thought it would be quite easy with all the streets in straight rows and numbered accordingly. The problem was that one had to be standing ready to leap off as soon as the tram stopped! The doors seemed to stay open only for a few seconds before one was swished on to the next stop. Eventually, I managed to disembark and walked back to the shopping street I wanted to look at.

After another night at the YWCA it was time to find my way to Kennedy Airport for my flight back to England. On the way home I reflected on the wonderful month I had just enjoyed. I also recalled that before my departure from the Radcliffe Infirmary the consultants had told me that, by law, the post of sister for the new Special-Care unit had to be advertised in the nursing press and that I must apply as soon as the advertisement appeared, as they were very keen that I should get the post.

Chapter 12

SETTING UP THE NEW SPECIAL-CARE UNIT

FOR CHILDREN AT THE RADCLIFFE INFIRMARY

Soon after I returned to England in 1970, the advertisement for a sister to be in charge of a new Special-Care unit for children having neonatal or cardiac surgery at the Radcliffe Infirmary, Oxford, appeared in the nursing magazines. I applied immediately and, to my great joy and excitement, I was chosen and asked to start as soon as possible.

The next three years were to be the most fulfilling and exhilarating of my life. First, I had a nursing post which I knew would be the pinnacle of my paediatric nursing career. Second, I met my husband David. Third, I married and had a child of my own. Fourth, my pay increased significantly. The different jigsaw pieces of my life were finally fitting into place.

For some time I had been annoyed at having to pay rent for my accommodation; also, I had given up hope of ever meeting the right man to marry. Thus, I decided, now that I was able to afford a small mortgage, to settle down and buy a small property of my own. I found just what I wanted in Woodstock, not far from Blenheim Palace; it was a small three-bedroom cottage which had been modernised. I fell in love with 3 Brook Hill as soon as I saw it.

My mother had recently bought a house on the coast opposite the Isle of Wight, and since it was smaller than the one she was selling in Winchester, there was surplus furniture. We each moved into our respective houses at about the same time. The week before I actually moved in I took possession and spent all of my off-duty hours painting the cottage throughout. Although my mother was busy with her own move, she found time to come and help me and revarnished all the wooden doors.

Soon after I had settled in I fulfilled another long-standing dream; I went a bit mad and bought a blue MG sports car with a soft top in exchange for my Mini. Of course the car was quite old, and I soon discovered that it used almost as much oil as petrol, but I was thrilled with it.

I spent the first month at the Radcliffe Infirmary equipping and setting up the new unit. There were two adjoining rooms in the new extension. The entrance was off the main surgical ward and led into the intermediary-care area, which could accommodate four beds, cots or incubators, depending on requirement, at any given time. Then there were sliding doors into the inner area, which was to be for most intensive care. Ideally, there would be one patient in this area at a time, but if emergency neonatal babies were admitted unexpectedly for surgery, it was quite possible to nurse two postoperatively.

Dr Richard Fordham was appointed anaesthetist in charge of the setting up and day-to-day running of the unit. He was a young, strong-minded and dedicated consultant with a particular interest in paediatrics; he was quietly spoken and had a caring and gentle way with children. I was glad we would be working together on this project.

One of the first things I had to choose was material for curtains and counterpanes. I was determined the unit should be a cheerful, homely and happy one. I chose a nursery design in bright colours for some of the curtains and a contrasting plain midnight blue. The unit had built-in wooden cupboards and work surfaces around the walls. It was quite a job thinking of all the things we might need for nursing these very sick postoperative children. When I first joined the unit, it was completely bare and empty, with no beds, lockers, incubators or even lights.

Our first task was to make long lists of the various equipment we felt would be needed in the unit. The lists of intensive-care equipment which I had seen in use in America and Canada came in very useful. Dr Fordham and I both wondered how on earth the hospital was going to afford everything. Then we heard that at the annual Children's Gift Service in Christ Church Cathedral, Oxford, monitors, incubators and special heaters were to be presented to the unit. These were paid for by money raised by the children of the Oxford Diocese, which each year chooses a different charity.

The selection of nurses for the unit went ahead, though I had no say in who was chosen. Seven really splendid girls came to form our first team on the unit; all but one were registered children's nurses. Julie, the one without the paediatric qualification, taught me much about immediate care, as she had worked for some time on Mr. Gunning's ward caring for adults after cardiac operations.

From the start we worked as a close team. Cardiac children were first admitted to the unit for investigations. Dr Pickering had by now returned from Toronto and was a consultant. He carried out all the cardiac catheterisations on the children who came into the unit. As soon as the unit was officially opened, any babies who were admitted to the hospital with serious neonatal congenital defects, such as tracheo-oesophageal fistula, imperforate anus, oesophageal atresia or exompholus, came straight into the Special-Care unit instead of the main surgical ward.

After setting up the unit, my main job was to train the nurses in intensive care. We were a mixed bunch: Julie, who was to become my senior staff nurse; Jan, who got married within about a year; Fran, who was Canadian; Aukje, who was from the Netherlands; Pippa, who was a very talented children's nurse; and Rosemary, the eldest, who was married with a family and working part-time. June, who had trained at the Radcliffe Infirmary, joined us a few months later.

I did not do any night duty, but the rest of the team worked in shifts to cover the twenty-four hours. One of my most difficult responsibilities was to work out the off duty fairly. As best as I could, I tried to accommodate all who requested special off-duty time, though obviously this was not always possible. It was paramount that we all got on and that there was a good, happy atmosphere.

Time and again I had to remind myself and my staff nurses that without surgery the children in our care would have died within a few months, that many cases had a very poor prognosis and that even with surgery many had only a fifty-fifty chance of survival. It could be very depressing, especially when we lost one or two children in a row. We had to support each other and be strong enough to help the families.

I still have a box of letters from parents who had children in the Special-Care unit. Here are two excerpts from these letters: "You have a happy little unit which makes the unhappy side of things so much less"; and "We were particularly touched by the way you treated [our child] as an individual, although he was so small, and not simply as a body needing medical attention. The sympathetic understanding and care of the nurses made the situation so much easier to bear."

During the first month or so that the unit was open we simply took the cardiac children for preoperative investigations. Mr Gunning, in preparation, went to the Toronto Children's Hospital to observe and work with Mr Mustard's cardiac surgical team. In fact, we were all getting heated up to start major cardiac surgery on children at the Radcliffe Infirmary.

It was suggested that I should take a two-week holiday before Mr Gunning returned. I decided to go skiing. At very short notice I contacted the Murison Small Chalet firm and was lucky enough to get the last vacancy in a chalet party at Wengen in Switzerland. There were about twelve of us, nearly all single and of roughly the same age group. I skied better and much more than I ever had before, or since. The weather and snow conditions were perfect. I acquired a fantastic tan and felt really fit. Our chalet girls gave us delicious home-cooked meals each evening. I even used my children's hostess experiences to dress up our chalet party as Indians in the fancy dress competitions at the nearby nightclub. We came in first out of ten groups!

We were approaching the end of our two-week holiday when I was told there was someone in the beginners' ski class who wished to meet me. Rather puzzled, I suggested he come to tea at the chalet.

The stranger was David. He asked me to join him for dinner that evening, the last night of my holiday. We went to a quiet little restaurant. I can remember little about the dinner, or what we ate, but I know we simply never stopped talking to each other, it was as if we had been close friends for years. I soon realised David was different from any man I had ever met. He was interesting and fun and full of humorous stories and little bits of useless but fascinating information. He had farmed, fished, shot and sailed, though now he was into antiques. He had obviously had a fairly wild past. The evening passed incredibly quickly. Later we joined David's friend, Edward, at a nightclub. Everything was perfect until David, in his usual honest way, told me he was married—with a family.

I returned to England the next day after a really wonderful fortnight's holiday. In my heart of hearts, I was very disappointed that David was married, but I told myself our relationship could have never been more than a holiday romance anyway, and I resolved to put him out of my mind and get on with my work in the unit. However, it was not as easy as that; we were like two magnets desperately seeking contact for several months. I did my best to avoid him. Throughout my time with the unit, he gave me tremendous support and encouragement. Gradually, I came to spend nearly all my days off with him, and we became very close.

Soon after I got back from Switzerland, Mr Gunning also returned. It was decided that we should now start major paediatric cardiac surgery. One of the first cases was a boy of six named Tony. He had a deficient valve which was restricting the blood flow from the heart to the lungs. Tony was a sensible little boy, and he did not look very ill on admission, but his condition prevented him from leading a normal, active life. Without an operation to repair the valve the prognosis was poor.

Dr Pickering, Dr Fordham and I explained all the equipment and procedures to Tony during the two days he was in the outer area of the unit prior to surgery. I took him into the intensive-care area and explained how it would be when he woke up. I assured him that his mother and father would be at his bedside, but there would be a lot of tubes and plasters attached to him; I also told him he must tell us if anything was hurting, as we could give him some medicine to make it better.

The evening before the operation, his mother read him a story and held his hand while he went to sleep. Parents of children in the unit could come in any time, night or day, and accommodation was also available for those wishing to stay overnight.

Tony's operation took three hours. A heart-lung machine was used whilst the actual valve was being repaired. This meant that Tony's heart stopped pumping and the machine circulated his blood. There were no complications during surgery or with his post operative nursing care. We were all jubilant. Tony recovered and was later able to live a normal life and play games at school.

Chapter 13
THE SPECIAL-CARE UNIT GOES FULL SPEED AHEAD

By June 1971, we were really busy. Our catchment area for babies requiring surgery for congenital defects was extensive; Banbury, Northampton, Abingdon, Aylesbury, Swindon and of course the Oxford area.

Our newborn baby was Paula; her parents lived in Cowley. Paula was born with tracheo-oesophageal fistula, that is, a hole between her feeding and breathing tubes. This is very serious defect and, if not detected at birth or before that baby has its first feed, can be fatal, as liquid passing through the mouth can go straight into the lungs, causing pneumonia.

Paula was transferred from the Oxford maternity ward to the Special-Care unit before she was twenty-four hours old. She was nursed in an incubator and within a few hours went to theatre for emergency surgery. Mr Gough was able to repair the fistula, and Paula returned to the Special-Care unit with a tracheostomy and a feeding tube in her stomach.

I felt a special closeness to this little baby as soon as I saw her and became too emotionally involved. She had every complication imaginable but was like a cat with nine lives. As Paula's parents never seemed able to bond with her and her mother was unable to hold her, I found myself giving Paula the love and affection that she needed so badly. I have often wondered whether we fought too hard. Might it not have been kinder to let her slip away during one of the very critical periods? But Paula had a strong will and survived against all odds.

During her good phases, Paula slept in a cot by my desk, in the outer part of the unit. Although she was unable to make the normal baby sounds because of her tracheostomy, she was extremely responsive and affectionate and had a wonderful smile. She stayed in the unit until she was eighteen months old. By this time she had put on a considerable amount of weight and seemed less susceptible to infections; her tracheostomy had been closed, and she was starting to make sounds. After much debate between nurses and doctors on the unit it was decided that Paula should move into the main ward, where her life would be more normal. She was still in there when I left the unit.

Once we got going with the major cardiac surgery, we had one regular operating day each week. Having had all their preoperative investigations, children were admitted from the waiting list. Many had already had surgery elsewhere to improve their circulation and to enable them to grow large enough for fully corrective surgery. Children were admitted two to three days before their operation so that they could settle in and to get to know the nurses, doctors and physiotherapists. This was a very important time, and I encourage my team to spend any spare minutes they had chatting with these children, playing with them or just cuddling them. A happy, confident child is much easier to nurse post-operative then a distressed, anxious one.

Christmas was a wonderful time on the unit. It was not practical, though, to decorate the inner intensive-care ward because of the risk of infection and the amount of equipment in use; besides, babies in incubators were too young to know about Christmas. But the other area looked really jolly with streamers, balloons and a little tree with coloured lights. On Christmas Day the doctors brought their own children in to see us, and I put a small present on our tree for each of them. In the window, I put a model crib scene to remind us all of the nativity.

We had a little dark-haired girl with us for my first Christmas on the unit. Jenny was five years old and came from a close-knit, loving family who lived in a country village outside Oxford. She was the youngest and the apple of her father's eye. Jenny, who had been a blue baby still had a poor colour and stunted fingers because of her poor circulation; but she also became breathless on the slightest exertion. Her father, however, had refused to give permission for a total correction of her Fallot's tetralogy, which was causing her breathing difficulty.

It had been explained to Jenny's parents that with so many defects in her heart she had a poor prognosis. They were also told that the operation would be risky and lengthy and that she would have only a fifty-fifty chance of a complete recovery. Jenny's mother had given permission, I think because she realised the operation was the child's only hope of an improved lifestyle. Eventually, after weeks of meetings with doctors, nurses and social workers, Jenny's father was persuaded to give his consent to the surgery.

Jenny, with large brown eyes, had a really beautiful face. On admission, she was painfully shy but not as withdrawn as she had been on her previous stay for cardiac catheterisation. Somehow it was even more important than usual that we succeed in helping this very sick child. This was one of the first total corrections that Mr Gunning had attempted from the unit.

Jenny received all the usual preoperative preparation. But this time I had compiled a detailed work list for the two staff nurses who would look after Jenny for at least the first four hours after she returned to the unit. They were called nurse 1 and nurse 2, so that this work list could be used after any open-heart operation.

Most of the observations were recorded every quarter of an hour by one nurse, while the other nurse recorded all intravenous intake, catheter output and drains. In this way each nurse knew exactly what she had to do and what she was responsible for.

Jenny's parents stayed in the visitor's room all day. Her mother and I accompanied Jenny to theatre, and we stayed in the anaesthetic room until she was fast asleep; it must have been around nine in the morning when we left her. The operation took all day. I kept in close touch with the theatre and with her parents.

The most critical and emotional stage of these operations was when the corrective surgery had been completed and the child's heart was reconnected to its own arteries and veins. When the heart-lung machine was stopped, everyone said a prayer, crossed his or her fingers and waited to see if the heart would start beating again.

Jenny's operation went according to plan, and at 4.00 I was asked to go and collect her from theatre. My two intensive-care staff nurses came with me. Dr Fordham looked after respiration whilst the two nurses and I carried all the various bottles, monitors and drains. The transportation of these children back to the unit was extremely tricky and had to be carried out with infinite care. It took about an hour to get Jenny settled back into the unit. When we were happy with her condition and comfort, I fetched her parents so that they could be with her when she woke up.

I quickly learnt how devastating it was for parents to see their child for the first time post operatively. Consequently, I would spend time explaining exactly what parents would see when they entered the room, and once there I told them what all the various tubes were for. Sometimes the children would be attached to a respirator for the first day or so in order to rest the heart as much as possible or because the lungs, not always fully expanded, were unable to oxygenate the body satisfactorily. Parents often found the respirator difficult to cope with, especially when the child woke up and was unable to talk because of the tracheostomy or intubation tube.

Jenny made a remarkable recovery, and after a few days her parents went home to the rest of the family and visited daily. But unfortunately, just when we were getting ready to discharge her, she spiked a temperature and was found to have a small wound abcess. It really was a blow, as she would have to have daily dressings and a course of antibiotic injections. This turn of events also meant she would have to stay in the unit for Christmas.

On Christmas morning Paula was there with a broad grin across her little face whilst two other toddlers were playing happily with the contents of their stockings. But Jenny was in her bed looking really miserable. Her family didn't have a car, and there was no public transport from their village on Christmas Day. I thought perhaps Radio Oxford could help. Without stopping to ask my superior's permission, I looked up the station's telephone number in the directory, called them and within minutes was connected to a very helpful man. I explained Jenny's predicament and asked if there was any way they could help. "Yes, of course," the man said and promised to send out a message after the next record.

Within an hour I received a telephone call to say a man who was alone for Christmas would be delighted to collect Jenny's family and bring them in to see her. Another volunteer, recently divorced and missing his own children badly, would come to the hospital at teatime and transport the family home again. I was excited and amazed. How easy it had been! Jenny and I did a little dance round the unit; it was wonderful to see her smiling again. Jenny is now married and has a healthy daughter of her own.

In January 1972, Reverend John Barton came to the hospital to be interviewed for the job of chaplain at the Radcliffe Infirmary. The matron telephoned me to say he would be coming to look round the Special-Care unit.

For some time I had felt I needed to acquire a stronger belief and inner strength for the work I was doing. Being sister of the paediatric intensive-care unit was extremely stressful and tiring, for so many people needed my support—the parents, the children themselves and my nurses. It was an enormous help to be able to go and see Reverend Barton at any time, especially just after I had to tell parents that their child had died on the operating table. I was frequently angry and upset, accusing God of not caring and letting these children die. Somehow John put things into perspective and encouraged me to go on. Later on John gave me and my new husband our first communion together in the Radcliffe Infirmary chapel.

Nearly all of the very sick newborn babies were christened at their parents' request before surgery. Some of the older cardiac children undergoing risky major surgery were also christened if they had not already been baptised as babies. With Reverend Barton's help, I bought a beautiful silver cross, bowl and spoon, which we used on these occasions.

I had often wondered what the children themselves thought about the unit. So when I decided to write this book I wrote to Nichola, and this is what she recalled:

In 1971 I was twelve years old and had a large ASD (hole between the atria of the heart) and a pulmonary stenosis (narrowing of the pulmonary artery). I had previously had thirteen operations in other hospitals.

I was admitted to the new Special-Care unit for final corrective surgery. The night before my operation, I sneaked out of bed to join a birthday party with the nurses and doctors and was given some cake. On the morning I was to have surgery I was given a premed injection into my right thigh; it was terribly painful, in fact, the worst part of my whole stay. Mum sat next to me and read me a fairy story until I fell asleep.

The next thing I remember is waking up after my operation and trying to pull off the oxygen mask. I did not like the smell of it. I was in the intensive-care room, which I had been shown the night before; there was only me and an incubator with a baby at the other end of the room. I was aware of all the tubes and drains and being restricted in my movements in the bed.

The doctor came and asked me what I felt like. I remember replying, "A marmite sandwich." I thought he meant what did I feel like eating. I was given a tiny marmite sandwich and was told to eat it slowly. I think it took about an hour to finish it.

The next day most of the drips, drains and cathethers were removed; the catheter was the most painful. After a couple of days I was moved back into the outer part of the unit, where there were four patients. I remember being cold and wet at night, because I was in an oxygen tent with a metal box full of ice at the back of my bed.

Mum was allowed to wash my long hair, and I was horrified at the amount of blood that came out when it was rinsed.

I remember two little babies in the unit with me; they were both terribly sick. After I got home Mum told me they had died.

I vividly remember Mum and Dad always being there throughout my stay, and although they didn't have much money, they always brought me a surprise. They never looked worried, but I know they must have been terrified. I am sure the fact that they were there had a great deal to do with my good recovery.

When she grew up and left school, Nichola trained as a nursery nurse. She said she was influenced by the nursery nurse on the unit at the time of her operation. She then became determined to go on and do training so that she could nurse sick children. Because of her history of congenital heart defects and surgery, no hospital would accept her for training. Eventually, after persistently applying to different hospitals, she did get accepted for an enrolled nurse's training. Nichola did extremely well and today is working as a senior nurse on a busy paediatric ward.

Whilst I was working on the Special-Care unit, it was suggested to me that I might write an article about paediatric intensive care after major cardiac surgery. So I had a go at it, and on 13 January 1972, my first article, entitled "Care of Children Undergoing Cardiac Surgery", was printed in the *Nursing Times*. The magazine included two photographs that I had taken in the unit. Of course I was absolutely delighted and decided to write a different article for the *Nursing Mirror*. This time I decided to describe Mr Mustard's operation, which I had watched in Toronto. Mr Gunning had performed the same operation on a child in our unit, and it had been successful, so I felt I was qualified to write something on the subject. This time Dr Pickering assisted me by providing some extremely good photographs to illustrate the article. It was entitled "Transposition of the Great Vessels" and was printed in the *Nursing Mirror* in September 1972.

All the doctors who worked with us were extremely dedicated and hardworking. Many a night, after a major cardiac operation, Dr Fordham would ask me to arrange for him to have a bed ready in a corner of the outer part of the unit so that he could be on very close call overnight. He usually stayed when a child was on the ventilator. It was not because he did not trust our nursing care but simply because many complications can occur when a child is on a ventilator, and the cause must be found and dealt with immediately so that no strain is put on the child's heart or lungs. Only an experienced paediatric anaesthetist can cope with such emergencies, and Dr Fordham was willing to spend the night on the unit so as to be there if the nurses needed him. I am sure our good success rate had a lot to do with his dedication.

My training at Great Ormond Street Hospital had a tremendous influence in the way I ran the Special-Care unit. When a child died, I always thought back to the time I had first experienced the death of a loved child and the sensitive and caring way the sister in charge had helped me. I tried to do the same for my staff nurses. There is no doubt at all that nurses looking after very sick children do get emotionally involved and that they would not be satisfactory paediatric nurses if they did not. But I now know, being a mother myself, that I could not have coped at the time if I had had a young family of my own at home. There is a certain point at which one must become controlled and detached in order to be able to help shocked and grieving parents. The paediatric nurse has a uniquely close relationship with these parents, or should have, and it is up to her to give as much support as possible.

Towards the end of 1972, my senior staff nurse, Julie, whom I knew and trusted well, asked to have a word with me in my office. I hadn't realised, until she told me, that I had become nearly impossible to work with. Thankfully, I had a senior staff nurse who was kind and brave enough to tell me the truth. Two years of stress on the Special-Care unit was taking its toll on me. Not only that, David had asked me to marry him. I was emotionally in a turmoil and, without realising it, had been taking all my worries out on the nurses.

Julie definitely did me a favour by being so frank and honest. I went home and had a good cry and a good think. In my heart I wanted to marry David and move on, so I decided to hand in my resignation, let my cottage in Woodstock and move to be nearer David in Shropshire. I have never regretted this mammoth decision.

Chapter 14
MARRIAGE AND A CHILD OF MY OWN

My last four weeks on the Special-Care unit were happy ones. Once I had decided to share my life with David, I was very much more relaxed. By this time, too, the unit was running smoothly. There was an excellent team of specialist paediatric nurses, and all staff members working on the unit had more confidence in their abilities. We had a really good run of cardiac and neonatal surgical successes.

Christmas on the unit that year was especially memorable. David came to Woodstock, and as I was on duty, he even came to see the unit on Christmas morning. It wasn't until some years later that I realised what an effort David's visit must have been for him; he hated anything to do with "blood and guts", as he called it.

On that Christmas morning, one of the very sick babies in intensive care had a cardiac arrest—a real emergency. David then saw the pressures I had been under, in addition to the importance of my unit and its experienced staff.

During the evening David and I had a wonderful Christmas dinner together at a hotel in Woodstock. He gave me a beautiful ruby-and-diamond ring, which fitted my finger exactly. This was a marvellous surprise on my last Christmas in Woodstock.

Soon after the New Year I had a leaving party at my cottage, and David came to help me entertain the guests. The only person unable to come was Alf Gunning, who was abroad at the time. The staff nurses gave me a cookery book. It was well known that I was not much of a cook, and they thought I might need some help with feeding David once we were married.

At last, in January 1973, I moved to Shropshire. For the first few months I worked as a part-time staff nurse on the children's ward at Copthorne Hospital, Shrewsbury. It was good to be so much nearer to David. He had bought a Victorian-terraced house in Bridgnorth and was busy modernising it. I set about making curtains for all the windows. We had great fun looking for furniture and planning our home together. Moreover, I enjoyed my part-time job. I had little responsibility, and I was still working with sick children. Also I met Gill, a physiotherapist who became a good friend and gave me my godson James.

In June 1973, David and I were married at the Chipping Norton Registry Office, my mother arranged a reception at the hotel in Woodstock, where David and I had eaten our Christmas dinner together. We spent the first night of our honeymoon at the Bull Hotel in Burford; then we called at Bridgnorth on our way to Scotland for a fishing honeymoon. David's dog, Bodger, a real Heinz 57 variety with a rough, black-and-white coat and bearded face, was supposed to be going into kennels while we were away, but he jumped into the boot of the car and refused to come out! We hadn't the heart to force him, so he came with us on our honeymoon.

On arrival at Perth, David still had no idea where in Scotland we were to stay.

David got into a conversation with a policeman, who turned out to be a very keen fisherman himself. Within a short space of time we were fixed up with hotel accommodations and salmon fishing for four days on the river Tay. Thus, in a hotel on the banks of the river we had a blissfully happy honeymoon. I was perfectly content to sit in the boat with David, Bodger and the ghillie whilst David fished for salmon.

We returned to Bridgnorth, relaxed and happy. I continued to work and enjoy my part-time job at Shrewsbury, and David and I settled down contentedly in our Victorian-terraced house. We both agreed that we would love to have a baby. I desperately hoped we would. I was thirty-seven, and David was nine years older.

In August 1973, two months after our wedding, we spent a week with David's younger sister and her family in Abersoch. I am almost certain that our son was conceived the same night as his little cousin. At any rate the two were born one week apart. I knew almost immediately that I was pregnant. I just felt different, but I kept it to myself until my suspicions were confirmed after six weeks by the doctor.

We were overjoyed. David already had three children from his first marriage, but it was my first experience with parenthood. I seemed to bloom and was incredibly healthy and happy throughout my pregnancy. But I discovered that although I was qualified and experienced as a children's nurse, because I had not done a midwifery training, I was quite ignorant about pregnancy. Moreover, because I was thirty-seven years old, I was in the category of "elderly primates". This meant I was put in the care of a consultant and was seen in an antenatal clinic at Wolverhampton about three times during the nine months.

All went smoothly until the end of the third month, when I was threatened with a miscarriage. Fortunately, Dr Michael was on call that night. He was out on a case when David telephoned, but his wife, a trained nurse, gave us excellent advice. I was to go straight to bed and remain as calm as possible. I had to stay in bed for three days, but luckily, everything settled down, and after a week I was back to living a normal life. I did, however, give up my part-time job on the children's ward. To fill in some of my spare time I joined a painting-for-pleasure class at our local adult education centre.

Our baby was due to be delivered just about a week after our first wedding anniversary in June. On 12 May 1974 I set off to gather moss in the country lanes about two miles from Bridgnorth. I wanted to get my hanging baskets planted before I went into the hospital. Not long after I had returned home, our son gave us warning that his arrival might be imminent. To my advantage, I had my case packed and everything ready. David telephoned the hospital, and we were told to go to Wolverhampton as soon as possible.

When I had been admitted and examined, to my dismay, I was told that although it seemed to be a false alarm, I must stay in the hospital until I went into labour properly. However, by the time David came the next evening I was getting regular labour pains, and by 10.00 our son was yelling his head off in my arms.

I was lucky enough to find breast feeding easy and pleasant. My son, whom David and I had named William was a tiny baby, weighing only five and a half pounds, but from the start he was strong and active.

My consultant knew that I was a Great Ormond Street nurse, and when I asked to stay in for the full ten days allowed for a first baby, he said I could, understanding that I wanted to get a good breast-feeding routine established before I went home.

Chapter 15

AN OVERWHELMING DISAPPOINTMENT

William's early childhood passed all too quickly. I have never before felt so content or fulfilled. Amusing and interesting, my son was a delight to look after. When he was three years old he started going to a local nursery several mornings a week. I missed him enormously, and although David and I had originally agreed to have just one child, I began to long for a brother or sister for William.

I was fortunate to become pregnant again within a few months. Everything progressed normally until at about the sixth month. During a routine checkup with the consultant at Wolverhampton, I was found to have a placenta previa. This means that the placenta would be delivered first, instead of after the baby's arrival. I was warned that there was a danger of a haemorrhage before full term. I should have taken this warning much more seriously.

David and I always went to Scotland in September for salmon fishing. With the baby due in November, we decided it would be wiser for me not to join the fishing party. I was to stay in Shropshire with William. David invited my mother to take my place.

On the day that my mother and David set off for Scotland, I thought I'd take William, now four, to the Dudley Zoo, which is about a half-hour drive from home. The zoo is situated on a hill. A path climbs fairly steeply, and there are different animals in cages to see on the way. I was incredibly fit and healthy. At times when William was tired, I wheeled him in the pushchair without realising that it might be unwise to exert so much energy. It was a happy day. I was sitting watching William on a child's roundabout when I suddenly felt a haemorrhage. The consultant had told me that if I did haemorrhage, I must get to the hospital in Wolverhampton as soon as possible.

It was difficult not to panic. I was on my own with William, a half-hour drive from home, and David and my mother were on the way to Scotland. The roundabout stopped, and William came running over to me. I knew I must stand up and walk some thirty yards to the ticket office. I told William he must be very grown-up and good, as I was not feeling well and might have to go to the hospital to have the baby.

At the ticket office I quickly explained the situation and was given a seat. An ambulance was called, and someone rang to ask my friend Joy to come and fetch William. In the middle of Sunday lunch, she dropped everything and set off immediately.

One of the worst moments of my life was when the ambulance arrived and I realised that William would be left for a while with total strangers. I was extremely frightened and felt quite alone on that ambulance trip. The police looked after William until Joy arrived to collect him from the police station. He remembers being shown inside police cars and being allowed to listen to mobile radios and sound car alarms.

The journey to Scotland took about six hours, so David didn't find out about my troubles until around five o'clock in the evening. As I was not critically ill, the doctor advised them not to return until the next day. I did feel very ill and scared and was relieved to see David and my mother again. For the next month I was on bed rest in the hospital to prevent any further haemorrhage and to enable my baby to grow before being delivered at full term. My mother looked after William and David at our house for the first week, then a friend named Liz took over until I eventually returned home. Liz had been a nanny before she married. She and her husband were on leave from a job in Saudi Arabia.

David came very evening to see me at the hospital. It was hoped that everything would settle down and the bleeding would stop. I was allowed to have a shower, but each time this brought on a haemorrhage, and I had to go back to bed rest. I began to worry about the health of my unborn baby. But after two scans, the doctors decided to wait and not do a Caesarean section until the baby was ready for delivery.

I knew the exact moment when my baby died. I had to keep a chart noting the times I felt the baby move or kick. These movements became less and less frequent, and then suddenly it was if there was a tremendous battle inside my body. I felt really strong kicks and then nothing more. A few hours later I had another scan. I have never felt so sad or disappointed. I was eight months pregnant and felt I knew Ben, my unborn child. I was quite unable to telephone David: it would have been too emotional. A great friend very kindly went round to see him.

The next day my stillborn baby was delivered by Caesarean operation. I had intended to see Ben after the operation. That morning, before I was taken to theatre, I made a tiny posy of flowers to put in my baby's hands, just as we used to do at Great Ormond Street, but shortly after I came round from the anaesthetic, the consultant came to see me. He had been shocked and surprised to find that my baby had so many congenital deformities. Some were rare ones, similar to those I had encountered in the Special-Care unit. None had shown up on scans. The consultant felt it would be wiser for me not to see the baby, and he also strongly advised me not to have any more children.

I was totally devastated. At last I understood how the mothers of babies who had died in the hospital unit must have suffered. Then came panic. Would Ben have a proper burial? It was a nightmare.

David put my mind at rest, and he made all arrangements. I didn't go to Ben's burial as I was still in the hospital, but I knew he was laid to rest in our little church-yard and that our vicar and David said prayers for him.

From this experience I learned firsthand how important it is for mothers of stillborn babies to be given as much help and reassurance as possible and that arrangements for burial or cremation must be discussed. To a mother a baby is a real, live being from conception. When things go wrong, she needs to grieve. William came to see me at the hospital every other day.

I did have a period of severe depression following the loss of our second son. But time is a great healer. In February 1979, David took William and me for a skiing holiday; we joined a couple of friends who had been regular skiing companions, and they were particularly kind and sympathetic to me. I returned home feeling refreshed and able to face the future.

Chapter 16
MY PLAYGROUPS

About three months after our holiday, William began full-time education at the local Catholic primary school. He settled in quickly and spent the next four years there. He made many friends and learnt the three Rs, arts and crafts and many other interesting subjects.

I missed William a great deal and found it hard to wait for him to come through the school gates at half past three. Always eager to tell me about his day, he was also ravenously hungry. I could never have been a full-time working mum and have missed, among other things, those daily chats on the way home from school. However, I soon realised that I wanted to have more contact with small children again. I knew we could not increase our own family after the devastating experience of losing Ben. But I did not want to continue nursing sick children. I needed to find something to do during term times and William's hours in school.

When I was a sister on the Special-Care unit in Oxford, I had occasional part-time jobs with an agency called the Oxford Aunts, where "aunts" helped in all kinds of emergencies or situations, like caring for children while mothers were working, ill or on holiday. "Aunts" also escorted children to airports or ships. Were there young mothers in the Bridgnorth area who would like to leave their baby or small child with a responsible person for a few hours while they went shopping, to the dentist, doctor or hairdresser or even to work? I decided to put this advertisement in the local paper: "Bridgnorth Aunt, Mary Aston, RSCN, SRN, is willing to look after small children in her own home for a few hours, in order to give their mothers some time off."

I received two fairly quick responses by telephone. The mother of a sixteen-month-old girl wanted to leave her child with me for a few hours one morning a week. The other call was from a mother whose third child, a boy of two, was hyper-active and difficult to cope with. She said she was desperately tired and would love one free morning a week.

In 1979, the rules for child minding were lax, until the Children's Act was passed. But if I was going to look after children in my home for payment, I decided I should get properly registered. So I approached the Shropshire Social Services and filled out the necessary forms. In due course, my house was inspected, and three months later I received the certificate saying I was a registered child minder.

Having interviewed the two prospective children with their mothers and after arranging the mornings when they would be in my care, I began a new career. It very soon became apparent that, although keen to leave their children with a child minder, at that time mothers did so with a slight feeling of guilt; but they were satisfied if they knew they were leaving their child in the care of a child minder who provided stimulating toys and activities in a happy home environment. So the "Mary

Aston" playgroup system was started.

Now in 1995, I am just completing my fifteenth year of running playgroups. The first children that attended are learning to drive and have taken their "A" levels. William has just left university with a degree. The years seem to have passed in a flash. I read the local newspaper each week to see if any of my pupils have shot goals for football teams, have been selected for swimming, tennis or cricket teams or have taken part in school plays.

My routine and organisation are just "different" from those of other groups. For one thing, I divide my children into three age groups, with the youngest on a Wednesday, starting at about two years and eight months. The three-year-olds come on a Thursday, and the eldest group of four-year-olds on a Monday. All the children play in my thirty-foot kitchen, which is attractively furnished and carpeted, for two-and-a-half-hour morning sessions.

I offer a wide assortment of constructional, educational and stimulating equipment for the children to play with. Each week, using cards, materials, paints and glue, we make something different the children can take home. Sometimes we make biscuits or cakes, which are always very popular. I help each child, as it is important to teach even very small children how to hold a paint brush correctly and to take a pride in their work.

During the morning we all sit down for a drink and a biscuit. Good manners are encouraged, and I find this a wonderful opportunity for conversation. If the weather is suitable, after our snack and a visit to the toilet, in Wellington boots and jackets we set off for a half-hour walk, either to the nearby park or to visit a neighbour's fish pond. On one occasion when we were all making a fuss of a friendly cat—only about fifty yards from the fish pond—I did not notice two of the boys leave the group and go on to the pool. Suddenly, there was a scream, and then a dripping wet Robbie got out of the water. Fortunately, the pool was shallow. I had taken children to see the fish for over ten years, and nothing like this had ever happened before. It was a lovely, sunny day, and after the initial shock, Robbie seemed quite unconcerned, so we all made a joke of it. We walked home quickly, and whilst my assistant amused the rest of the group, I gave Robbie a warm foam bath and dressed him in dry clothes. The incident was entered into my accident records and, of course, the whole tale had to be recounted to his mother. She just laughed and said, "Oh, no, Robbie, not again!" Apparently, he had done the same thing the previous week in his own pool at home. We all agreed he had better learn to swim as quickly as possible.

I have never found it necessary to advertise my groups. They became known by word of mouth or personal recommendation, and I have always had a waiting list. Local doctors and health visitors frequently referred children whom they felt would benefit from my Great Ormond Street sick children's training.

Over the years, I have had several children with special problems. Danny had Stickler's Syndrome. It is very rare, and I had never heard of it before. He was diagnosed and for the first years of his life was treated at Great Ormond Street Hospital. He first came to my playgroup at the age of two and a half years and spent a session on his own with me each week. Danny had poor sight and wore thick plastic lenses in each eye. He also had a hearing aid in each ear; these were attached to a small battery box he wore in a harness on his chest.

From the start, Danny was an active, happy little boy and was most affectionate. Within a few months I was able to let him join the youngest session. He moved up through each age group, and it became obvious he was intelligent and would need special education. When he was nearly five years old Danny left and went to a special school for blind and deaf children. Some years later his mother, who is musical, discovered that Danny had perfect pitch. He started to have piano lessons and later learned the violin. Now at seventeen, Danny has nine GCSEs and is at present studying for three "A" levels in music, physics and maths.

Tom was another little boy who, as a baby, survived all the odds. He was a patient of Mr Gough at the Radcliffe Infirmary, where I had been a sister. Tom had started life with a tracheo-oesophageal fistula, a hole between his breathing and feeding tubes. Mr Gough was able to repair the fistula, and after long periods of hospitalisation, Tom was well enough to stay at home. When he was about two years old, the family moved to a small town close to Bridgnorth. Tom's mother had heard about my playgroups from a medical practice.

Tom was a delicate, thin, pale little boy with carrot-red hair. At first his mother was very nervous of leaving him. Tom settled quickly, and though he was never unhappy at playgroup, he was painfully shy and had difficulty holding a pencil or paintbrush. This was mostly due to poor coordination and lack of confidence, but as the weeks passed, he improved and became more relaxed. Tom has since had to return to the hospital for more major operations on his throat. But when I last saw him, he was a tall, sturdy lad in his last year at boarding school and was studying for "A" levels.

Sally was born with spinal muscular atrophy (SMA). She had a marvellously supportive family, loving and intelligent parents and two sets of devoted grandparents. Their great concern was that Sally should have as normal a life as possible, though they realised she would never walk on her own.

Sally was born at the same time as another little girl in Bridgnorth, and their mothers became great friends. When the children were about eighteen months old, Sally's mother telephoned to make enquiries about my playgroups and to put the two little girls' names on my waiting list. There was a noticeable pause over the line. The mother wondered if I would still be willing to have her daughter in my playgroup. When I said I'd be delighted to have Sally, I could sense her mother's relief.

Sally was about two years and eight months when she started coming to the playgroup. She was angelic to look at, with short, sleek, straight blonde hair and a fringe. Obviously, she had to be carried about, but she had her own special chair to support her back. Later she would bring a frame to stand in at the table for painting, drawing and other creative activities. Always bright and cheerful, Sally was a popular member of the group. Her best friend, almost like a second mother, passed toys just out of reach and generally looked after Sally. If the group had musical games, I danced with her in my arms. Her father was clever with his hands and adapted their house to enable Sally to be as independent as possible.

At the age of five Sally entered a national Christmas card design competition organised by the Jennifer Trust for SMA. Her design, a robin wearing a bobble hat, won the competition and became a Christmas card which was sold all over the country to help other children with spinal muscular atrophy. Sally had already shown great courage and determination. She now has a younger sister whom she adores. Sally copes very well in a normal primary school, and her own electric buggy gives her independence. Her best friend moved away from Bridgnorth, but Sally is still surrounded by a circle of caring, friendly children and takes part in all kinds of local activities. She loves swimming and is a Brownie.

The children I remember very well are the ones who were really difficult at first. Over the years there have been several who threw awful temper tantrums when their mothers left them. This kind of behaviour was quite different from that of a child who sobbed and was genuinely unhappy when the mother left the room. The child who throws a real tantrum is usually very bright: these children are trying for attention. They might kick, spit, scream or even scratch. When I was less experienced, I tried all kinds of ways to calm these children but discovered such attention made them worse. Now I let them lie on the floor, and I pretend to ignore them for a while. As the shouting and temper tantrum decrease, I leave various toys within reach. I pretend to take no notice and occupy myself close by, secretly watching reactions. Usually, the child suddenly cheers up and starts to play normally. Treated this way, I find they hardly ever have another tantrum when they arrive at playgroup. Sometimes I have found it helps if a child brings a small toy of his own to show me when he arrives. This distraction can help to prevent a tantrum.

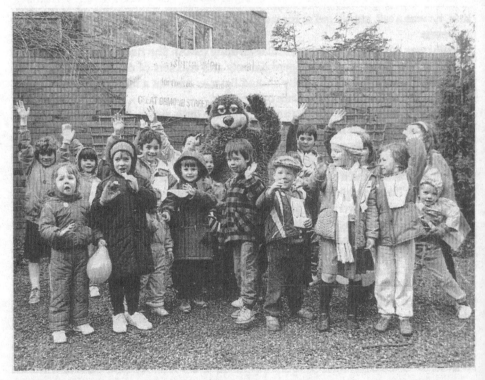

Children's sponsored walk in aid of "The Wishing Well Appeal" for Great Ormond Street Hospital. William is in the bear costume.

Children can react in other ways besides tantrums. Some will be very quiet and not want to join in activities or play with others. Sometimes little chatter boxes at home will not even speak to us when they first start coming to playgroup. Gradually, over a few weeks, however, these children grow in confidence and come out of their shells.

At Christmas we have a party. As there is little space, I can only invite one parent, usually the mother. The room is decorated with balloons and festive cards, and rows of chairs are arranged for the mums at one end. At 11.45 there is great excitement when children of all ages arrive dressed in party clothes. While the mothers have a glass of wine, their offspring entertain us with a selection of songs accompanied by finger or hand actions. Finally, Henly, our window cleaner who recently retired, appears dressed as Father Christmas, as he has done every year since I started my playgroups. Each year he gets better and better at his Santa Claus act. Although he is a very well-known character in the Bridgnorth High Street, none of the children has yet guessed his real identity. He distributes a present to each child and chats with each one as he or she comes forward. Before Henly leaves we join in singing his favourite carol, "Away in a Manger". Then the adults enjoy homemade mince pies, and the children share iced Christmas-tree biscuits. The party only lasts about an hour, but it is always a great success, and the children, each trailing a balloon, go home in high spirits.

By the time the children leave to start school, nearly all are able to write and recognise their own name, count to ten and know most of the alphabet. Each child in my four-year-old group has a workbook with a picture on the front: a robin or a mouse and so on. Each week they use them for a different project I have prepared for them. When the work is completed, they receive a star for effort.

I have had children from several large families attend my playgroups. I am always amazed at how completely individual and different each child in a family is, and yet there is always a strong family identity. There is no doubt in my mind that the way children behave very much depends on the treatment and amount of loving care they receive at home. This becomes very obvious when three or four children come from the same family, for I find they all behave very much the same; for example, they are all either bad mannered, very affectionate, precocious, undisciplined, etc.

I can honestly say that I have loved every playgroup session and feel very fortunate to have played a part in the early formative years of so many children. For the fifteen years that I have been running playgroups I could not have coped without Mrs Murdo. She not only cleans the house but is a great favourite with all the children. In an emergency or if my assistant is ill, Mrs Murdo has often helped with the sessions. The children have started a tradition of calling her in for coffee when it is drink time. There are three doors that go into the kitchen, and the children love to guess and point at the door through which they think she is going to enter. It is a very simple game, handed down from group to group over the years. Mrs Murdo is very much a part of the playgroup scene in my house. I have also been very lucky with my dedicated assistants. Now that I am nearing retirement, I know how much I will miss children coming to my home three times a week.

Chapter 17
CHILDREN FUND-RAISING FOR CHILDREN

A few years after I had begun running playgroups, in 1985, Great Ormond Street Hospital for Sick Children launched its "Wishing Well Appeal". The famous hospital was desperately short of funds and needed to raise money to carry out its splendid plans to reconstruct and modernise the building.

I was in an extremely good position to raise money for a cause so close to my heart. A larger number of parents had, by then, enrolled their children in my playgroups, and many of these parents owned businesses in Bridgnorth or were professional people. What I needed was to think of an interesting fund-raising event and organise it.

I decided on a children's sponsored walk. In Bridgnorth there is an old church, St Leonard's, which is surrounded by a close, mostly used by residents. Because there is no through traffic, it seemed the ideal place for children to walk in safety.

First I had to find a local business willing to provide several hundred sponsor forms. I designed one and needed copies made. Bridgnorth Enterprise Garage agreed to help. This was a good start. Next, I asked the police to give permission for a sponsored walk in St Leonard's Close. A few days later I received a letter giving me the go-ahead and the information that two volunteer special officers would be available to assist with traffic problems. I was also advised to notify all the residents in the close of my intentions and to request that cars be parked elsewhere that afternoon.

Marshals of some kind would be needed to count and record the number of laps each child completed, so I asked the local Girl Guide companies for volunteers. They were very keen to help, and I had enough girls to act as marshals and work in the hall and pin a number on each child before the walk started. A travel agency in the town gave me hundreds of old cards they were just about to throw out. On these I printed a number of each child taking part.

It was important to have some special attraction during the walk. Eventually, I had an inspiration. I had taken my son, William, and some of his friends to Alton Towers Theme Park the previous holiday. Here, men dressed up in life-sized Disneyland costumes and mingled with the visitors. We enjoyed most a big, furry bear. I wrote to Alton Towers and explained that I was organising a children's sponsored walk in aid of the Wishing Well Appeal and asked if it would be possible to borrow the bear costume. They agreed to loan the costume if I could collect it and promise to return it in good condition. At this time, William was about eleven years old. With his talent for acting and his good rapport with children, he would be the ideal person to dress up as the bear, but I wondered if he would have the courage. He agreed to do it.

About three weeks before the event, I visited each primary school in Bridgnorth, and whenever possible, I talked to the head. I left sponsor forms at all the schools and also at our local leisure centre and post offices. Forms were also delivered to each family in the town whose children had attended my playgroups.

In order to be able to use collection tins during the walk, I had to become a registered charity collector for Great Ormond Street Hospital, so I did. Several parents offered to hold a tin at strategic positions round the close. Finally, the editor of our local newspaper agreed to print a short account of the proposed walk, giving venues where sponsor forms could be collected.

During the week before the walk I found myself constantly going over all the details. I had no idea how many children would turn up on the day, for everywhere I went, whether it was in the town, at our local supermarket or at the leisure centre, I asked any children I met if they had a sponsor form, told them about the walk and encouraged them to take part.

On the actual day, the weather was fairly good; the sun wasn't shining, but it was not raining. The walk was due to start at 2.00 P.M. The volunteer special officers set up bollards and cleared the close of cars. With the help of the Boy Scouts we prepared the hall; as it was their building, their mothers had offered to serve tea and soft drinks after the walk; the Cubs did their bit by blowing up hundreds of balloons to be distributed at the end of the walk. By 1.30 a short queue began to form outside the hall, and at 1.45 we opened the doors and began to pin numbers on the children, who then took up positions behind the starting ribbon. I had asked Danny, a former Great Ormond Street patient, and also one of my playgroup pupils, to cut the ribbon when the church clock struck 2.00.

Soon it became obvious that a great number of Bridgnorth families had decided to take part in the walk. It had been made clear on the sponsor forms that smaller children could be accompanied by parents and babies could be carried. The maximum number of laps to be attempted was twenty.

While everyone was collecting and the spectators took up positions, William played a great part by walking round in the bear costume, stopping now and again to shake a paw with a child. They loved him, and it was just the added attraction we needed. Although he got terribly hot inside the fur material, William still kept going throughout the walk.

After signing their form, each child was given a Great Ormond Street badge and a balloon; many of the families ended the afternoon by visiting the scout hut for well-earned refreshments. When all the money was counted, I was delighted to be able to send a cheque for £1,500 to the Wishing Well Appeal. It had all been very worthwhile.

A few years later, in 1989, to celebrate the tenth year of my playgroups, I decided to have a swimming party for all past and present pupils. Just at that time, Bridgnorth Cottage Hospital was under threat of closure. The manager of Bridgnorth Enterprise Garage, who had assisted me with the walk for the Wishing Well Appeal, pledged sufficient money to keep the hospital open for two years. At the same time there was an appeal for funds for the hospital. Everyone in the Bridgnorth area was asked to do whatever they could to help. So instead of just having a swimming party for the ten-year celebration, we would have a sponsored swim followed by a tea party.

When I visited the *Bridgnorth Journal* office to ask if they would advertise the swim, a local wealthy businessman overheard my conversation and asked if he could help. He gave me a cheque for fifty pounds. Thus, all overhead expenses—renting the local swimming pool, with attendant lifesavers, and the hire of a hall for the tea party—would be covered.

I persuaded friends to come and count the widths of the pool each child swam. Each friend would sit on a chair at the edge of the pool, and a marker on the other side of the pool would indicate a channel for the swimmer to stay in. A maximum of fifty widths was decided on. Non-swimmers, who had to be accompanied by an adult, could do one or two widths in the shallow end. These children wore armbands and rings. I was stationed at the entrance to collect sponsor forms. Again, I was amazed at the number of children who took part and was especially delighted to see so many of my former pupils.

At the end of the swim, we all went into the hall, where there was a wonderful spread of food. I had asked all the girls to bring a plate of sweet things, either cakes or biscuits, and the boys to bring savouries, such as crisps, sausages, or sandwiches. Some of my playgroup parents had arranged it all on a buffet table. At the end of the party, in order to applaud the children's accomplishments and to give me a chance to see each child individually, I handed out the sponsor forms and announced the number of widths each child had swum. I then collected all the sponsor money and was delighted to be able to hand in a cheque for £340 to the hospital.

Now, in 1995, I am slowly winding down my playgroups. By next year I shall be running only one short pre-playgroup session a week. However, I am determined to keep in touch with local children. For example, I will continue to organise the junior church group in our parish. This group of children over three years old, which meets once a month, gives me another opportunity for contact with small children.

I realise how fortunate I am to have been surrounded by children throughout my life.